JOHN COOKSON

JOHN CRAMMER

BERNARD HEINE

The Use of Drugs in Psychiatry

in Psychiatry

Fourth Edition

GASKELL

First published 1978
Second edition 1982
Third edition 1991
Fourth edition 1993

Gaskell is an imprint of the Royal College of Psychiatrists,
17 Belgrave Square, London SW1

British Library Cataloguing-in-Publication Data
A catalogue record for this book is available from the
British Library.
ISBN 0-902241-63-X

Distributed in North America
by American Psychiatric Press, Inc.
ISBN 0-88048-626-0

Publication of this book was made possible by the kind
support of Roche Products Limited.

Printed by Bell & Bain Limited, Glasgow.

Contents

Part III: Drug list

Acknowledgements

About 15 years ago, Dr Brian Barraclough first had the idea of this book and recruited John Crammer and Bernard Heine to help create it. Together they planned what it should contain: to be a practical pocket book that the beginner could consult in clinic or ward. They wrote their selected topics separately, exchanged typescripts and met on several occasions to debate content and expression. It was Brian Barraclough, above all, who emphasised the need for clarity and simplicity. The result was published in 1978, and a new edition in 1982.

At the time of the third edition Dr Barraclough was not able to take part in the final re-writing and editing. It was realised then that any subsequent edition would require a contribution from a younger active clinician versed in neuropharmacology. John Cookson has taken on this role and written new sections and, with Bernard Heine, revised others.

Earlier editions were greatly helped by Drs Michael Best, John Corbett, M. Faulk, G. Fenton, J. Grimshaw, M. Lader, C. Nunn, E. H. Reynolds, and Eric Taylor. For their advice on the new edition we are grateful to Drs J. Herzberg, M. Farrell and E. Taylor, and to Ms Paula Wilkinson. We have not necessarily adopted their views. However, any errors, distortion or important omissions are ours alone: we hope, of course, that there are none of substance.

Finally, our thanks go to Mrs Helena Warren and Mrs Daphne Green for so ably producing an ordered typescript and disk.

How to use this book

This is a practical book, for use in surgery, clinic or ward. It advises when and how to use medication to help people with behavioural and psychological disturbances, whether these are primary mental illnesses or secondary to physical illness. Drug prescriptions are described in the context of the general management of the individual patient. Where possible, treatments are based on securely established fact, otherwise they represent our own experience and what we teach as good practice. It is not necessarily the only successful way of doing things, but one we can recommend in the present state of knowledge. But it is based on our belief that taking pains over the choice, introduction and dose schedule of drugs results in better therapeutic results and less toxicity.

In the past, many psychiatrists have been prepared to take great trouble over their psychotherapeutic handling of patients, but used drugs in a fast, indifferent, rule-of-thumb way. They have sometimes been frightened of proper doses or persisting for long enough with medical treatment, and have not learned that understanding chemotherapy can improve the outcome for their patients. We believe that psychological treatment, informal or formal, must often be combined with drug treatment, in a balanced way, to relieve and to cure.

The book is divided into three sections. The first is the general elementary introduction to the neurobiological background and to psychological and social factors to be borne in mind in good prescribing. It can be read as a whole, or in parts, at any time. The second is a series of short essays on the different psychiatric situations and syndromes usually met, and the third an account of all the drugs currently available in Britain for psychiatric treatment. These sections work together and have a good deal of cross-referencing. In everyday use one dips into the book by looking up an individual drug through the index of trade and approved names; or uses the symptom index to see what the book says about treatment of a particular symptom or syndrome. Or one can take the patient's diagnosis, read the appropriate management essay and look up the mentioned drugs in the drug list.

While, simply for information, we give the names of all available drugs we give details about only a few. In each group we give one at length which we regard as typical of the group and well established, and in general to be most highly recommended, and follow it with shorter entries on some others of the same group which we regard as useful. When describing side-effects we try to name the most common and most important first, the lesser ones later; and we do not list all the side-effects ever reported because to do so is to raise unnecessary fears and to blur the impact of the important with excessive information about the rare. The doses described here are intended to be consistent with those in the *British National Formulary* and the manufacturers' data sheets, but refer to the treatment of adults who are not elderly. In treating the elderly, lower doses are always required.

This is an elementary book, for beginners in psychiatry, medical students, general practitioners and casualty officers, and perhaps helpful also to nurses, social workers and clinical psychologists. It is not intended as a consultant's guide, or as a review of progress in psychopharmacology. Brain structure, neurotransmitters and receptors are described, focusing on aspects which seem of most relevance to the drugs in current use. At present, biological science helps us to understand something of how drugs work and their side-effects, but casts little light on the underlying pathophysiology of mental illness.

We should use the drugs we do on the basis of systematic empirical experience with many patients of different types, and their careful clinical study, and not because of any hypotheses about the nature of mental illness.

Our book reports some of this experience. In recognition of the importance of new drugs for improved treatments and the role of clinicians in studying these we have introduced a chapter on the development of new drugs. The book is not intended primarily as a text of psycho-pharmacology but as one which describes how drug therapy fits into the wider context of psychiatric treatment. Everyday practice is our touchstone.

Abbreviations used

ACh	Acetylcholine
ADH	Antidiuretic hormone, vasopressin
c-AMP	Cyclic-adenosine monophosphate
COMT	Catechol-ortho-methyl transferase
DA	Dopamine
D-	Dopamine receptor subtype
DOPA	Dihydroxyphenylalanine
GABA	Gamma-amino butyric acid
H-	Histamine receptor subtype
5-HT	5-hydroxytryptamine, serotonin
5-HIAA	5-hydroxyindole acetic acid
HVA	Homovanillic acid
M-	Acetylcholine muscarinic receptor subtype
MAOI	Monoamine oxidase inhibitor
MARI	Monoamine reuptake inhibitor
MHPG	Methoxy-hydroxyphenylglycol
NA	Noradrenaline
RIMA	Reversible inhibitor of monoamine oxidase
m-RNA	Messenger ribonucleic acid
SSRI	Serotonin-specific reuptake inhibitor
TCA	Tricyclic antidepressant
TRH	Thyrotrophin releasing hormone
TSH	Thyroid stimulating hormone
V-	Vasopressin receptor subtype

Part I. The background to good prescribing

1 Prescribing for psychiatric patients

The use of drugs in psychiatry differs from their use in other branches of medicine in three important ways.

Psychotropic drugs suppress psychological symptoms and morbid behaviour which has no known physical pathology. How drugs do this is unknown. The justification for their use is based entirely on clinical experience. The contrast with the knowledge of disease pathology and drug action which supports drug use in general medicine is striking.

Mental illness interferes with insight, the capacity to view an illness with objectivity and agree the correct treatment. Mental illness may even prevent recognition that an illness exists at all. Impairment of insight, a topic barely relevant to general medical patients, often interferes with understanding the point of medication and adherence to a plan of treatment.

Every individual has a social existence, and disturbances in behaviour and feelings can have enormous repercussions on family, friends and workmates. Therefore, treatment of individuals may harm or help those around them and this must always be borne in mind

How does this affect the prescribing of psychotropic drugs? Firstly, psychotropic drugs suppress symptoms and are used to tide the patient over until the brain dysfunction, whatever it may be, remits. After some months of use, when a drug such as lithium or chlorpromazine is stopped, the symptoms originally abolished may reappear.

Psychiatric diagnoses depend on groups of symptoms occurring together and have no basis in pathology or aetiology. So labels such as schizophrenia or neurotic

4 The background to good prescribing

depression cannot imply a single pathological entity or a particular chemotherapy. Although many symptoms of schizophrenia are often suppressed by chlorpromazine, this is not an antischizophrenic drug, and to think so will create prescribing error and poor outcomes for some patients.

Chemotherapy is based on trial and error, on empirical experience, and it is sometimes justifiable to use a psychotropic drug in novel circumstances. This is how effective knowledge has so far been built up, and will be extended. But a consequence is that follow-up of the patient to discover what exactly happened after one week, one month, even one year on the drug is more important in psychiatry than in general medicine. This is how useful personal experience, and general knowledge, grow.

Secondly, patients may find it difficult to believe they are ill, or that a physical agent can help them solve what may appear to them as an emotional problem, or face what seems to them some unpleasant reality. They will need psychological handling to accept a drug. The doctor has to engender confidence and assess how much of the patient's behaviour is personality and how much the disability of illness. For example, was he always a timid, anxious, hypochondriacal person; has illness made him suspicious of everyone, or forgetful? The answers determine what the doctor says and does in explaining the illness and what can be done about it and how a drug or medicine may play a part.

Similarly, the doctor's success with the patient may be supported or undermined by the relatives and by other helpers who may or may not share the doctor's views about mental illness and the role of medication.

Not only personality, morbid and premorbid, but attitudes and lifestyle must be taken into account. Someone who is worried about chemical pollution of the environment or the risks of drug addiction may need education and psychotherapeutic persuasion to accept a psychotropic drug, and understanding the individual's particular difficulties is helpful. The regular drinker of alcohol will not take medicine which he thinks goes poorly with alcohol, unless special work is done to harmonise therapy with social life through some acceptable compromise. A man who always takes cheese sandwiches to work will not want an MAOI, which interacts with it. Someone on the night shift will not want a drug three times during the day. Very frequently, therefore, psychiatric prescribing is much more than writing the names and doses of drugs on a sheet of paper. It involves a transaction in which the doctor accepts and neutralises the patient's fears, and a choice of drug and a timing of doses to suit the patient's daily routine.

Thirdly, it is always useful to ask oneself, "who has sent this patient to the clinic?", "why is this patient in hospital?", meaning "who has urged or insisted that the patient seek medical help?", because very often relations or workmates, social workers or lawyers or other outside professionals have prompted referral and are expecting some change in the patient. Treatment has therefore to be directed towards them, too. For example, a person who is getting up in the middle of the night and going downstairs to wander about may not complain of insomnia or daytime fatigue, but may be alarming his relatives by his unpredictability, and a hypnotic prescribed to the patient may be primarily to soothe them. Of course, the relatives should be given some explanation of the nature of the illness, and what to expect from it and from the treatment plan, but the drug prescription may take them into account, too.

Psychiatric illness may impair a sufferer's self-awareness and knowledge of the impression they make on others, and may also diminish the care they take of themselves and their appreciation of their own interests. Doctors must therefore take on a greater responsibility for their patients, a quasi-parental role, if they are to serve them well, and serve the community in which they live. General practitioners in particular quite commonly leave it to patients to come back to them if they are dissatisfied or not doing well. This will often not do for psychiatric patients; the doctor must give them a definite follow-up appointment (and even if it is not kept, check why not, and make another) for a day or two hence, or a week or two, to see whether the prescription has resulted in any changes. It may be important to ask a relative to come to the appointment too (or to phone in some report). The patient may not have taken the medicine, or may say it has done no good, whereas the relative may have noted a striking improvement; or it may have produced new symptoms and the doctor should learn of this. The telephone can also be useful for the follow-up of patients who have difficulty travelling or are staying at a distance.

An important part of the art of practice is knowing when to follow up, how often and for how long, and in what ways. Psychiatric illness in particular is often chronic even though fluctuating in severity or punctuated by long remissions. It is especially important to have some rational plan of when and how to follow it through, and to ask members of the family or community, particularly those close to the patient, from time to time to give their impressions of progress.

With psychiatric patients one quite often needs to make a balanced judgement between opposing considerations. Thus psychiatric illness sometimes impairs common sense and self-care. If left to care for themselves they may fail to do so. How far in respect for the individual and the right to self-determination should one let a patient go, even perhaps to allowing suicide, or should one intervene at some point and complete some kind of treatment? Suppose a young schizophrenic is unable to work or look after himself and is willing to have treatment, but the only drug which helps him back to some semblance of normality carries some risk of an irreversible side-effect: should one prescribe it or not? A woman with a history of several manic–depressive breakdowns is successfully kept free of further breakdowns with lithium or carbamazepine, but wants to become pregnant. The drugs may cause foetal malformation: should she stop them forthwith, and run the risk of further breakdowns (suicidal depression, or reckless excitement, perhaps) or let the foetus carry the risk of cardiac or neurological anomaly? We believe each case must be considered individually to balance the various desires and risks against one another, in the context of known reported risks.

In the next chapters, there are explanations of how drug interactions can occur. In psychiatry some of these inter-actions are beneficial, some adverse, and they may be overlooked. An example of an apparent beneficial interaction is between amitriptyline and lithium which together may relieve severe depressive illness not well controlled by either drug alone. Often two or more drugs have to be prescribed at the same time, and interaction may occur in absorption and metabolism, or at sites within the nervous system. The persistence of metabolites and other effects after a drug has been stopped may influence the actions of the next drug taken.

The art of prescribing includes the following considerations:

(a) the symptoms to be targeted in the short and the long term
(b) age, physical health and circumstances
(c) drugs already taken, including home remedies such as cough cures
(d) the effectiveness, and otherwise, of previous drug treatments
(e) personality and lifestyle
(f) the social setting
(g) the choice of actual drugs; size and schedule of dose
(h) when to review outcome and who should help report it
(i) the role of the community psychiatric nurse and the general practitioner in providing medication and monitoring progress.

Not infrequently the answers to these considerations conflict and do not lead to a logical, ideal drug treatment. For example, a sedative antidepressant may impair driving ability and a commercial driving licence can be suspended, with temporary loss of employment and income. A life with regular depot injections required to prevent a relapse of schizophrenia entails side-effects which would be unacceptable in other circumstances.

Decisions from conflicting evidence are common in medicine. They are best made after discussion with the patient and the patient's relatives or others who have a legitimate interest. Ultimately, however, the doctor, because of his or her technical knowledge and experience, must decide, acting in the best interests of the patient.

The following chapters in Part I deal with relevant pharmaceutical, pharmacological and metabolic aspects of drugs. Chapter 5, "Clinical practice", covers some psychological and social points, and under the heading "Unexpected results" discusses what to do when treatment unexpectedly fails, or new symptoms appear, and includes idiosyncrasies and the investigation of drug interactions.

2   The metabolism of drugs

Pharmacology

When a patient takes a drug prescribed by a doctor the effects are both pharmacological and psychological. The latter arise because human beings are responsive to their doctors, to their changing social environment, and to their own sensations and expectations, and can be influenced by what the doctor says and does. It is always necessary to try to disentangle the pharmacological from the psychological response in treatment, so as to make balanced decisions about the role of drugs.

In this chapter and the one which follows we are concerned with the physical factors which determine the pharmacological response in the patient. Some concern the way in which the drug in a medicine enters the body and travels in the circulation reaching a well protected brain, others the way it alters the functional balance between different groups of nerve cells in the brain. Modern psychotropic drugs have been known for only 40 years and their discovery has been partly accidental and partly by scientific planning and determination. How to use them safely and effectively has been found by the hard practical experience of treating thousands of patients, made more precise by the pharmaceutical and metabolic considerations described briefly below. In recent years, more has become known about the mechanisms by which drugs act. Unfortunately, little is known about the basic neurochemical abnormalities underlying mental illness. Thus neurotransmitter studies and theories, although intellectually appealing, are of more relevance to understanding how drugs work than to understanding the illnesses. Careful detailed observation of what drugs do, singly and in combination, in human beings suffering with different clinical conditions, remains the line of progress in therapeutics.

Terminology

It will be useful to explain a number of terms used in clinical pharmacology.

Pharmacokinetics is the study of all the factors which determine the concentration of the drug at its site of action – "what the body does to the drug".

Pharmacodynamics, on the other hand, is the study of the mechanisms by which a drug exerts its actions – "what the drug does to the body".

It is the former we are concerned with in this chapter.

Bioavailability is the extent to which the drug reaches the brain when taken by a patient orally as opposed to the same quantity of drug given intravenously.

In trying to understand the relation between size of dose, concentration in the blood and duration of clinical effect, a simple model is often used. The body is assumed to be a single vessel of fluid in which the drug will rapidly disperse, and the *volume of distribution* of a drug is the volume of the imaginary vessel as shown by the diluted plasma level to which the drug falls shortly after its administration and rapid absorption. Elimination of most drugs follows *exponential* or *first-order kinetics*, that is, a constant fraction of the whole in the body is eliminated per unit of time, independent of the actual concentration of the drug. This corresponds to an exponential decline in concentration. But a few (e.g. phenytoin, alcohol) are eliminated by rather feeble processes, by enzymes present in such small amounts that the concentration of drug quickly saturates them. When the enzymes are working thus at maximum pitch, a constant steady quantity of drug is eliminated per unit of time, whatever the body load. This slower process is one of *zero-order kinetics* and the concentration in the blood declines linearly. The *elimination half-time*, the time taken to eliminate half the drug administered, is a convenient measure of persistence in the body, which will affect the frequency of dosing. Another measure, the *plasma half-life*, indicates how long it takes for the concentration of drug in the plasma to decline to half its previous level. Another is the *clearance*, the fraction of the total volume of distribution emptied, theoretically, of all drug in unit time.

Measurement of plasma concentrations of a drug at various times after a single intravenous dose can show the elimination kinetics, the volume of distribution and plasma half-life, and thereby indicates what dose, repeated in what frequency, should be used to achieve any chemical concentration in the body fluids at a certain time. They are used to establish how to prescribe a drug, especially if new.

From knowledge of a drug's half-life, one can predict how long it will take for a steady state to be reached after regular dosing commences. Thus, after the passage of two half-lives, the concentration of drug in the blood will have reached 75% of the eventual steady-state level; after five half-lives it will have reached almost 97% of the steady state. Thus, for a drug such as haloperidol with a half-life of 18 hours, the steady state will have been almost reached after about 90 hours, or four days. A depot drug such as haloperidol decanoate has an average half-life of about three weeks and during regular dosing the steady state will not be approached until 15 weeks have passed. Under circumstances where the half-life is very long, it makes sense to give a loading dose or more frequent initial doses to reach the desired steady-state level more quickly, and then reduce the frequency of dosing to maintain it. It should be noted that the time taken to reach the steady state is the same whatever the frequency of dosing, although the absolute level of the steady state will be higher with more frequent doses or larger doses.

Tolerance is said to have occurred when the same drug

effect can only be obtained by increasing the dose. This is sometimes due to pharmacokinetic reasons, the drug being metabolised more quickly when the body has been exposed to it longer. Alternatively, tolerance may represent an adaptation to the action of the drug so that a high concentration is needed to bring about the same effect.

Tachyphylaxis is the rapid development of tolerance after only two to three doses; this is most often due to desensitisation of the drug receptors.

Dependence is where there are physical or psychological symptoms on attempted discontinuation of the drug.

Drug addiction is where much time is spent on drug-seeking and drug-taking behaviour, with physical and psychological symptoms on withdrawal.

Bioavailability

Not all tablets or capsules disintegrate easily in the stomach, and not all suspensions have particles of the right size for easy solution or absorption. Different preparations or brands of the same drug do not always yield the same amount of drug in the patient. Oral preparations do not keep indefinitely, and many preparations have a limited shelf-life, deteriorating after their 'use-by' date. Intramuscular injections of the same preparation of the drug do not always give the same effect. Choice of muscle, needle position, depth of injection, tissue trauma and blood flow through the muscle influence the speed and completeness of absorption. Inactivity and poor circulation, notably in the chronic schizophrenic, the elderly, and the physically ill, may delay uptake.

A tablet is not all active drug, but contains an excipient which binds together and adds bulk to the tablet and is covered with a coating, often coloured. An injection has a vehicle; a syrup may have a solvent, a stabiliser and a preservative. Occasionally these supposedly inert substances have unwanted effects, producing for example an allergic reaction. (Changing to another brand of the same drug, made up differently, may then avoid these bad effects.) Defects in bioavailability may sometimes explain the failure of a drug to produce the intended response.

Absorption

Some drugs are absorbed from the stomach, others only from a part of the intestine. Delayed gastric emptying may slow the action of intestinally absorbed drugs if taken before a meal, when the pylorus is shut. Some drugs, lithium carbonate, for instance, are gastric irritants and best taken with some food. The pH of gastric and intestinal contents, intestinal hurry or delay, the nature of the diet and its digestion, may influence absorption. A partial gastrectomy, malabsorption syndromes, and diarrhoea may alter the speed and completeness with which a drug enters the portal circulation from the gut.

Drugs absorbed from the gastrointestinal tract must pass through the mucosa into the portal circulation and through the liver, and some are at once partly destroyed in the mucosa and liver ('first-pass metabolism', which may be substantial) before distribution to the rest of the body. Others – diazepam, some antidepressants and antipsychotics for instance – have therapeutically active metabolites produced in the liver. In contrast, drugs given intravenously, intramuscularly, or sublingually are distributed to lung and then to brain and body with a smaller fraction to the liver. By these routes the brain gets a bigger share of the drug than from the same oral dose. Since liquids or syrups are more quickly absorbed than the contents of tablets, they too may give rather more drug to the brain. In fact, diazepam taken as a liquid by mouth is effective more quickly than the same dose given by intramuscular injection. How a drug is to be taken (by mouth?), in what form (age and brand of tablet?), and how often (once a day?), often need to be considered.

Metabolism

The liver is the chief site of drug metabolism, but lung, gut wall, kidney and placenta also attack drugs and so do the microflora of the gut (Fig. 1). Liver metabolism occurs via the cytochrome P450 series of enzymes. The activity of this system is at its highest in childhood and declines with

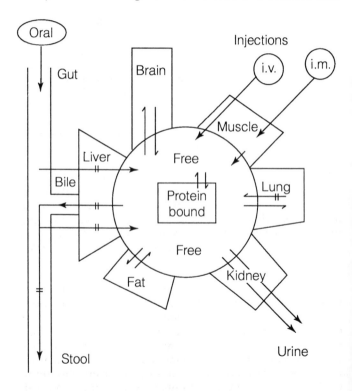

Fig.1   A diagram of drug metabolism. The circle represents the blood, arrows indicate drug movement, and parallel lines on arrow shaft indicate drug metabolism

age from the early teens. Liver enzymes that metabolise drugs are reliably increased in quantity, or 'induced', over a week or more by many substances – tobacco smoke, alcohol, phenytoin, and some psychotropic drugs (barbiturates, carbamazepine, phenothiazines, orphenadrine). Heavy drinkers and smokers, epileptics and other chronic drug users may therefore need bigger doses of a psychotropic drug than usual if the brain is to get its share. Chlorpromazine and carbamazepine stimulate the liver enzymes that destroy them and other drugs. Their psychotropic effects sometimes seem to wear off after about two weeks of use because additional enzymes become active and the drug is destroyed more quickly. A higher dose is then needed. In contrast, patients with congestive cardiac failure or other causes of limited hepatic blood flow; liver damage; babies with underdeveloped liver function; and the elderly with diminished hepatic performance require smaller doses of many psychotropic drugs than the norm for their body weight.

Certain steroids, particularly progestogens which are used in oral contraceptives, inhibit drug metabolism. A female patient taken off 'the pill' may then require more psychotropic drugs as her metabolism increases. Pregnant women, with their raised progesterone levels, metabolise drugs less effectively. Drugs to be continued through pregnancy may need to be reduced in dose if they are subject to metabolic destruction, but increased again after labour.

Drug metabolism is sometimes considered in two phases. Phase I involves enzymatic oxidation or reduction, hydroxylation, demethylation and hydrolysis; all produce metabolites which are more water soluble, so that a greater proportion of them can be excreted by the kidney. Sometimes these metabolites are pharmacologically more active than the parent compound, but more often they are inert. Phase II is the conversion of phase I metabolites to conjugates by acetylation, sulphation or conjugation with glucuronic acid; these are very water-soluble and excreted by the kidney. Phase I metabolism is reduced with ageing but phase II tends to be maintained even in the elderly.

Thus, drugs which are metabolised mainly by phase II, such as oxazepam, do not accumulate to a much greater extent in the elderly. In addition to the decline in liver enzymes, including the P450 system, in the elderly, the liver metabolism is also more likely to be diminished because of concurrent physical illnesses and the use of medication of other kinds.

Certain liver enzymes are particularly important in relation to psychotropic drugs. Thus the hydroxylase CYP II D6 plays an important part in the metabolism of tricyclic antidepressants. About 6% of Caucasians have low levels of this enzyme and are slow metabolisers of these drugs. These can be detected by their slow metabolism of debrisoquine or dextromethorphan. Similarly, a proportion of individuals have low levels of acetylase; this results in them being slow acetylators of drugs, including phenelzine. These are autosomal recessive traits. Some drugs inhibit the hydroxylase enzymes – for instance phenothiazines, fluoxetine and paroxetine – leading to increases in the level of tricyclic antidepressants by up to four times.

Entero-hepatic circulation

Drugs of larger molecular size and their metabolites are secreted by the liver into the bile and periodically emptied into the gut from the gall bladder, some to be reabsorbed into the blood. This entero-hepatic circulation of drugs results in a reserve of drug and metabolites remaining in the bile and gut contents, only some passing out in the faeces. Further, metabolites inactivated by hepatic oxidation may be reactivated by chemical reduction through the activity of intestinal microflora. Reactivated drugs then reappear in the circulation and prolong the pharmacological action. Drugs excreted mainly in the bile and faeces therefore take longer to clear from the body than those excreted in the urine. The normality or 'health' of a patient's microflora may influence what happens.

Fat solubility

Many drugs are highly soluble in body fat; the brain being composed largely of lipids takes up a lot of such drugs. When a drug is first circulating it rapidly enters the brain because of its high blood supply, but then if it is lipid-soluble it is taken up extensively by the adipose tissue of the body resulting in it being rapidly withdrawn from the brain again. Thus the drug is shared unequally between the body and the brain, the body getting most of it. A fat body gets an even larger share so that the brain gets less. A child of four has a brain of almost adult size which results in the brain getting a larger share of a dose than an adult brain would. Thus a lipid-soluble drug has a short activity half-life (in the brain) but a long elimination half-life. The short-acting barbiturates are examples of such drugs, as are some benzodiazepines such as lorazepam.

Renal excretion

Some drugs and their metabolites are excreted almost entirely in the urine; lithium is an example. Others are excreted partly in the urine, partly in the faeces. Thirty per cent of imipramine and only 10% of thioridazine are lost through the kidneys. Good renal function is essential for clearing many drugs and their metabolites from the body. Poor blood flow through the kidney, as in cardiac failure, or in renal disease such as chronic nephritis, or normally in the infant under one year old, may result in partial or complete failure to clear a drug. Normal doses then have the effect of an overdose. The extreme case is prescribing during renal failure treated by dialysis where the drug is only removed periodically in the dialysate, and has to be prescribed accordingly. The glomerular filtration rate declines slowly from the age of 30 and the renal clearance of drugs falls off after the age of 60.

Urinary excretion of drugs that are weak bases or weak acids depends on the urine pH, which may vary with diet and exercise. Conditions that favour salt formation also favour drug excretion. Thus a weak base such as amphetamine is excreted more rapidly if the urine is strongly acid, since it then forms salts which are not reabsorbed; but if the urine is markedly alkaline, the free un-ionized base diffuses out of the renal tubules back into the blood, and drug action on the brain is prolonged. Conversely, the excretion of weak acids such as barbiturates or salicylates can be increased by making the urine alkaline. The urine can be made acid with doses of ammonium chloride, or alkaline with sodium bicarbonate or potassium citrate.

Drugs in the blood

Since samples of circulating blood are easily drawn, measurement of the amount of the drug in the blood is a simple approach to the question of how much drug is reaching the sensitive areas of the brain – provided a sensitive and specific method exists for analysis of that drug. It is then possible to correlate the therapeutic and side-effects of the drug with its plasma concentration, provided: (a) the clinical effect follows soon after the drug reaches the brain; (b) it is due directly to the drug and not to some metabolite; and (c) the drug–brain receptor interaction is reversible (for most monoamine oxidase inhibitors it is not).

Thus for phenytoin and for lithium it is possible to find plasma concentrations associated with beneficial effects, and higher concentrations associated with adverse or toxic effects. These concentrations are similar but not identical in different individuals, which gives rise to the idea of a therapeutic range of values for a given population of patients. Low lithium concentrations have had little effect in treating groups of manic patients. As the lithium concentrations are raised above 0.7 mmol/l different patients respond as higher concentrations are achieved, but raising the level above 1.4 mmol/l has not produced any further benefits and toxic signs appear. Under these circumstances the therapeutic range of lithium for the treatment of mania is said to be 0.7–1.4 mmol/l, which means that the vast majority of patients who respond will be expected to do so on doses producing a plasma level in this range. But one particular individual may only do well at the top of the range, while a second recovers on 0.8 mmol/l, and a third may require 1.0 mmol/l.

For some antidepressants, plasma levels of the drug and its active metabolites can be measured, and approximate therapeutic ranges are known. This is done most commonly for amitriptyline and its metabolite nortriptyline. Nortriptyline itself is unusual in that blood concentrations above a certain level, about 150 ng/ml, are associated with a lack of response or side-effects. There is said to be a 'therapeutic window' between 50–150 ng/ml.

Phenothiazines are metabolised extensively and some metabolites are active. No clear relationships have been found between the drug levels for individual phenothiazines and clinical response. Haloperidol, on the other hand, is metabolised more simply and although its main metabolite, reduced haloperidol, may be active, a relationship has been claimed between haloperidol level and therapeutic response in schizophrenia, with blood levels between 5–30 ng/ml. There is some evidence that blood levels greater than this are associated with a poorer clinical response. In practice, blood levels are used clinically only for monitoring lithium, anticonvulsants (including carbamazepine and valproate), and occasionally amitriptyline and imipramine levels. One difficulty is that the clinical response (e.g. relief of depression) follows 10 days or more after the establishment of the drug level. What is happening in this time, and how is it related to the quantities of drug arriving over 10 days? (See page 198.)

Individual patients differ considerably in how they absorb and metabolise the same dose of a single drug. For instance, in a group all given 100 mg amitriptyline daily on the same schedule, there is at least a tenfold difference between the lowest and the highest individual plasma level obtained. For drugs such as chlorpromazine which induce liver enzymes, the variability between individuals is even greater. These differences are partly genetic but also reflect age, previous and concurrent drug therapy, and physical health. It was therefore hoped that drug measurements would provide a guide in deciding clinical doses for the individual, but this has not on the whole proved possible.

Plasma measurements, of course, reveal whether a patient has taken the prescribed drug (though not necessarily in the doses proposed), but they are an expensive way of testing adherence. They have been useful in studying drug toxicity (when linked to abnormally high plasma concentrations of the drug), and they are valuable in the discovery of drug interactions. For example, when chlorpromazine is added to a steady treatment with imipramine, the plasma concentrations of imipramine and desipramine rise almost at once to much higher levels. This is due to the competitive inhibition in the liver of imipramine metabolism by chlorpromazine, an interaction first discovered by plasma measurements. Many examples are now known where one drug inhibits the metabolism of another, or alternatively speeds up its destruction – for instance carbamazepine lowering haloperidol levels by as much as 60% – and blood measurements have been important in the discovery. Assays are therefore valuable in the analysis of unusual or unexpected drug responses.

There are two very important points to remember when interpreting measurements of plasma concentration of drugs. The first is that a blood sample is taken at a moment in time, and the measurement, therefore, applies only to that moment, like a snapshot. Other times of day might yield other values. Therefore, when taking a blood sample always mark the exact time it was drawn, and when comparing samples on different days try always to take them at the same time of day, and always avoid times soon after the actual taking of drug doses. With lithium this is particularly important because lithium is rapidly absorbed, and the plasma level rises rapidly in the next four hours and then falls away exponentially; blood for clinically useful lithium measurements should be drawn between 8–16 hours, preferably 12 hours, after the previous dose.

The second point is that with most drugs (but not lithium), the plasma proteins modify the values the laboratory returns. Most drugs circulate only partly dissolved freely in the plasma water and pharmacologically active; they are largely (80–95%) bound reversibly to plasma proteins, especially albumin, and this fraction is pharmacologically inactive. The laboratory reports the total drug in the plasma, free plus protein-bound, and unfortunately the latter is subject to hidden changes. If the plasma albumin is low, as in liver disease, the protein-bound drug will be low and the total concentration will be low, but the pharmacological action will be the same because the free drug concentration is the same. Or the albumin may be normal but its binding capacity for the drug being measured may be low, either because of competitive interference from another drug (very important when using two or more anticonvulsants, for instance carbamazepine with valproate or phenytoin) or because of metabolic interference – the binding is altered in uraemia, diabetes, ketosis, and starvation. Or the binding proteins itself can be increased in some chronic inflammatory conditions (Crohn's disease) or after trauma or surgery, and then bound drug will be high, total drug level high, yet free drug perhaps only just adequate. So total plasma drug concentrations offer many pitfalls, and are not quite the excellent guide to drug therapy that was first hoped.

Babies and drugs

Many drugs cross the placenta. The baby of a mother taking lithium may be born with hypothyroidism caused by the lithium; a morphine-dependent woman may produce a drug-dependent infant. With some drugs the main risk may be to cause an anomaly of development, which occurs chiefly in the first three months of foetal life, when anatomy is decided, and not thereafter. In deciding whether or not to give such drugs during pregnancy the stage of pregnancy is clearly important, but also it is necessary to weigh the pros and cons of treatment for both mother and for foetus, and not just for one of them.

Drugs also appear in breast milk, in proportion to their free concentration (not bound to protein, or total) in the maternal circulating plasma. Therefore, drugs like phenothiazines and tricyclics which are mostly protein-bound are of little import, but lithium, which is free, can matter. These considerations may contraindicate breast-feeding, unless the maternal drug can reasonably be stopped. Infants in the first year of life have poor renal and hepatic function so that clearance of drugs such as diazepam is slow at this time.

If a woman has to take drugs during pregnancy, remember that renal blood flow (and hence urinary excretion) increases at this time, but that the increased progesterone secretion suppresses hepatic metabolism of drugs. Drug dosage may need to be adjusted in the light of those facts, and readjusted after delivery.

Drug interactions

The simultaneous prescription of more than one drug is often necessary. However, drugs may interfere with each other's absorption from the gut, binding in the plasma, excretion in the urine, metabolism in the liver and effects in the brain. Some examples illustrate the point. Carbamazepine, like barbiturates, stimulates liver enzymes that destroy imipramine, haloperidol, phenytoin and other drugs, and may reduce the clinical effects of these drugs. Monoamine oxidase inhibitors block phenytoin metabolism and may cause phenytoin toxicity. Orphenadrine stimulates the liver enzymes that destroy chlorpromazine, diminishing

the levels of chlorpromazine, as well as interacting in the
brain to diminish its effects on the extrapyramidal system.
In contrast, chlorpromazine, fluvoxamine, fluoxetine and
paroxetine prevent the liver metabolism of imipramine.
Fluvoxamine slows the elimination of drugs metabolised
by oxidation in the liver including warfarin, phenytoin,
theophylline and propranolol. The doses of these drugs
should be lowered when prescribing fluvoxamine.

3   Drugs in the brain

The brain consists of a complex array of neurones, grouped into nuclei separated by axonal tracts supported by glial cells, and protected from the circulation by the blood–brain barrier; this barrier is permeable to fat-soluble compounds but only selectively to larger or highly charged molecules.

The past 30 years has seen an enormous increase in knowledge of cellular function in the brain. But this has led to only a modest increase, mostly speculative, in understanding the pathophysiology of mental illness. There is, however, a clearer understanding of the mechanisms of actions of psychotropic drugs. Unfortunately, this does not extend far beyond the primary site of action. We still know little about the more delayed changes that result from drug action, although these are more relevant to the slow changes seen in clinical conditions.

Much of our knowledge springs from the discovery of individual neurotransmitters, their synthesis, pathways and receptors. Much remains to be learned about how each neurotransmitter and its neurones interact with others. Also the more recently discovered neuropeptides are less amenable to pharmacological interventions, but are probably very important.

In this chapter we will consider individual transmitters that are known to be relevant to understanding drug action. Their synthesis, neuronal pathways, and receptors will be summarised.

Receptors

Receptors are the peptide structures to which drugs attach, and which initiate their effects. They consist of a recognition site and an effector. The effector undergoes a change in structure which leads to, for instance, the activation of an enzyme or the opening of an ionic channel. A drug which attaches to the receptor and activates the effector is called an 'agonist'; these are usually related structurally to the natural transmitter. A drug which attaches to the receptor and produces no activation is called an 'antagonist', because its occupancy of the receptor prevents the agonist or the transmitter from working. The interaction of most drugs with receptors is reversible, and a competitive antagonism occurs, in which a higher concentration of the agonist can displace the antagonist and produce an effect. Generally an agonist needs only to occupy a small fraction of the total number of receptors to produce a large effect, because there are 'spare receptors'.

As the dose of the drug increases, the quantity bound to the receptor increases in a hyperbolic manner towards a saturation level. When the relationship between the concentration of an agonist and the response is plotted on a logarithmic scale, an S-shaped log dose-response curve is observed. In the presence of a competitive antagonist this curve is shifted to the right in a parallel manner (see Fig. 2).

The dose-ratio, between the new concentration and the original concentration required to produce a given response, is related to the proportion of receptors occupied by the antagonist – the 'occupancy' – by a simple formula; dose-ratio $= 100/(100\text{-}P)$, where P is the percentage of receptors occupied. When 75% of receptors are occupied, the dose-ratio is 4; if 95% are occupied, the dose-ratio is 20.

This method has been used to determine receptor occupancy by antipsychotic drugs using positron emission tomographic (PET) scanning (see p. 234). At some peripheral synapses, such as the neuromuscular junction, there is a

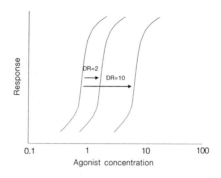

Fig.2   Shift to right in log dose-response curve for an agonist alone and in the presence of an antagonist at two concentrations producing dose ratios (DRs) of 2 and 10

'safety factor', so that a large proportion of receptors have to be occupied, perhaps 80%, before transmission fails. However, if there is no safety factor, and the log dose-response curve is steep, then a small occupancy will produce a large reduction in response. Transmitter pathways in the brain are resilient; during exposure to drugs, compensatory changes occur. For instance, in the presence of an antagonist the pre-synaptic neurone may – because of feedback inhibition – synthesise and release an increased amount of transmitter. The metabolites are then detected in increased quantities in the cerebrospinal fluid (CSF). Over the course of a week or more the post-synaptic neurones whose receptors are blocked will respond by synthesising more receptors – 'up-regulation' – akin to the phenomenon of 'denervation hypersensitivity' which follows transection of a peripheral nerve.

On the other hand, exposure to agonist causes two processes of reduced sensitivity. Firstly, there is a rapid 'desensitisation' resulting from a change in the structure on the activated receptor to one which is quiescent. Secondly, there is a reduced synthesis or 'down-regulation' of the number of receptors.

This resilience means there is also a 'safety factor' in brain pathways. Thus symptoms of Parkinsonism do not develop until some 70% of dopamine (DA) neurones in the substantia nigra have degenerated, or until 70% of the DA receptors in the basal ganglia are occupied by antipsychotic drugs in young adults (see below).

Receptors can be identified by 'labelling' them with antagonists containing a radioactive atom. If these 'ligands' are specific for a particular type of receptor, they can be used to measure the quantity of that receptor and its distribution in the brain. Receptors can then be classified according to the transmitter or agonist, the antagonist, and the type of effect. More recently, receptors have been identified from the RNA which synthesises them. Since the RNA can be cloned it is easier to study than the receptor itself and can provide the amino acid sequence of the receptor. Most receptors are localised on the surface of the cell in the membrane; but steroid and thyroid hormones interact with receptors that are intracellular.

Cell-surface receptors are of two main classes. Class I receptors are ligand-gated ionic channels. Their activation leads to a rapid transient increase in membrane permeability. This causes excitation or inhibition of the post-synaptic membrane. Examples are ACh nicotinic receptors (excitatory) and GABA-A receptors (inhibitory). These receptors consist of four subunits surrounding a 'channel' in the membrane. Binding of the agonist opens the channel.

Class II receptors produce slower responses involving so-called G-proteins which bind to the intracellular portion of the receptor and activate a second messenger. These receptors consist of a long peptide chain with seven subunits within the membrane and a long intracellular loop which binds the G-protein. Various second messengers may then be activated or inhibited including adenylate cyclase (producing c-AMP, leading to the phosphorylation of other enzymes), activation of phosphoinositide turnover and calcium release, the conversion of arachidonic acid to prostaglandins, leukotrienes and other active compounds, and indirect activation of ion channels.

Dopamine

Tyrosine is converted by tyrosine hydroxylase to L-dopa (dihydroxyphenylanine) which is decarboxylated to dopamine (DA). Tyrosine hydroxylase is the rate-limiting enzyme, and synthesis of DA can be increased by administering L-dopa. DA is stored in vesicles and released by nerve impulses. Released DA is taken back into the nerve ending by an active reuptake process. A small portion is also metabolised by MAO (monoamine oxidase) and COMT (catechol-ortho-methyl transferase), the main metabolite being HVA (homovanillic acid).

There are three main DA pathways in the brain.

(a) The *nigrostriatal pathway* which runs from the substantia nigra to the caudate-putamen in the corpus striatum. This pathway is important in involuntary muscle control including stereotypies. Degeneration of the pathway leads to Parkinson's disease.

(b) The *mesolimbic pathway,* from an area of the mid-brain close to the substantia nigra, projects into the 'limbic' areas of the brain. The limbic system is a collection of structures which lie along the medial surface of the brain, especially the temporal lobe. The essential components are the hippocampal complex, amygdala, cingulate gyrus, entorhinal cortex, septal nuclei and nucleus accumbens. There is a mesocortical pathway to the limbic cortex – the medio-frontal, cingulate and entorhinal cortex. The pathway to the nucleus accumbens is important in drive-orientated behaviour and locomotor activation; this tract will support self-stimulation by implanted electrodes, and DA injected into the nucleus accumbens causes increased locomotor activity. The meso-prefrontal DA pathway is activated by stress. It is also postulated to be underdeveloped in schizophrenia.

(c) The *short DA-neurone pathway*. Neurones in the hypothalamus include those secreting DA to the pituitary portal blood supply to inhibit the release of prolactin. Short DA neurones exist also in the 'area postrema' close to the vomiting centre.

DA receptors occur post-synaptically in these areas. Also, with the exception of the mesocortical neurones, the other long DA neurones have inhibitory pre-synaptic 'autoreceptors'; stimulation of autoreceptors inhibits, and blockade increases transmitter release. Thus, antipsychotic drugs lead initially to an increased firing rate of nigrostriatal and mesolimbic, but not mesocortical DA neurones. During long-term treatment the increased firing subsides and the former neurones become quiescent or inactivated (see p. 138).

DA receptors are of two main types, D-1 and D-2. The D-1 type stimulates adenylate cyclase and c-AMP as a second messenger. The D-2 type is not so linked. Subtypes of these exist and are differentiated by their antagonists and their location, a matter which has become important in understanding the actions of antipsychotic drugs (see p. 234). Thus D-3 and D-4, subtypes of D-2, are more common in the limbic areas than in the caudate-putamen, where other D-2 receptors predominate. In particular, D-3 receptors are common in the nucleus accumbens as well as D-2 receptors, but not in the pituitary; D-4 receptors are common in the amygdala and frontal cortex. D-5 is a subtype of D-1, present in the hippocampus.

Acetylcholine

Acetylcholine (ACh) is synthesised from choline and acetyl coenzyme A by choline acetyl transferase. Choline is the rate-limiting factor in synthesis but not in release. ACh is stored in vesicles and released by nerve impulses. Within the synaptic cleft it is inactivated by choline esterase. A reuptake process carries choline back into the nerve ending. Choline esterase is inhibited by physostigmine and by organophosphorus compounds which are used as insecticides.

Cholinergic neurones are widely distributed. They are inter-neurones in the caudate-putamen which receive an inhibitory input from the nigrostriatal DA pathway. There are two major ACh pathways, one from the basal forebrain (including the nucleus basalis of Meinert) projecting to the cerebral cortex and other parts of the forebrain. This includes the septal-hippocampal projection which is involved in memory. The second is from the mid-brain to the thalamus and to the pontine reticular formation.

ACh is thought to play an important part in short-term memory, and in arousal and cortical activation. Degeneration of cholinergic forebrain neurones (and other neurones) occurs in Alzheimer's disease, although the post-synaptic receptors are preserved.

ACh receptors are of two main types, nicotinic and muscarinic. Those in the brain are mainly muscarinic, and at least five subtypes exist (M 1–5). They are linked to G-proteins and a variety of second messengers. Atropine is the classical antagonist of M-receptors, blocking all subtypes. Many antidepressant and antipsychotic drugs block these receptors, especially in high doses.

Noradrenaline

Noradrenaline (NA) is synthesised from the amino acids tyrosine and phenylalanine, converted by tyrosine hydroxylase to L-dopa, by decarboxylase to DA, and by DA beta-hydroxylase to NA.

It is stored in granules in the nerve terminals which, in NA neurones, run diffusely for several centimetres, each containing several thousand terminal varicosities with granules. The rate-limiting step is tyrosine hydroxylase whose action is subject to feedback inhibition. The release of NA is regulated not only by impulse flow, but by pre-synaptic receptors including autoreceptors and opiate receptors. This interaction with opiate receptors means that, during opiate withdrawal, NA neurones are activated with increased release of NA. In some neurones NA co-exists with neuropeptides whose release augments the action of NA.

Released NA is taken back into the cell by a reuptake mechanism. A small proportion is inactivated by COMT and MAO-A. The main metabolite of brain NA is methoxy-hydroxyphenylglycol (MHPG), which is measurable in CSF and urine.

NA neurones have their cell bodies in the mid-brain. The largest group is in the locus coeruleus in the pons. Axons from these neurones send extensive branches to the forebrain, including the cerebral cortex, hypothalamus and cerebellar cortex. A second group is more loosely localised and supplies the amygdala and septum.

NA is thought to play an important role in the sleep/wake cycle, reinforcement, learning and affect. Locus coeruleus neurones are activated by unexpected sensory events. Severe stress causes an increased turnover of NA in the brain.

NA receptors are subdivided into alpha and beta types. Alpha-1 and beta receptors are mainly post-synaptic, alpha-2 receptors are both pre- and post-synaptic. Beta receptors are subdivided into beta-1, -2, and -3; all are linked to adenylate cyclase but sensitive to different antagonists (see p. 32).

5-Hydroxytryptamine

5-Hydroxytryptamine (serotonin, 5-HT), an indoleamine, is synthesised from the amino acid L-tryptophan, converted by tryptophan hydroxylase to 5-hydroxytryptophan, and by a decarboxylase to 5-HT. Synthesis and release can be altered by the availability of L-tryptophan in the diet which competes with other neutral amino acids for transport into the brain.

Release occurs by nerve impulses and is modulated by the pre-synaptic receptors. After release, 5-HT is inactivated by a powerful reuptake mechanism. A small proportion is broken down by MAO to 5-HIAA (5-hydroxyindole acetic acid) which appears in the CSF.

The cell bodies of 5-HT neurones are restricted to clusters in the midline (raphé) region of the pons and brainstem. There are also a small number of cells in the locus coeruleus and in the area postrema. The more rostral cell groups send axons with extensive innervation to the forebrain, including the limbic system, and an extensive diffuse innervation of the cerebral cortex. More caudal neurones supply the medulla and spinal cord. 5-HT has both excitatory and inhibitory effects. The neurones discharge rhythmically and they exert a simultaneous modulatory effect in diverse brain regions. The firing frequency is higher during alertness and reduced during sleep.

Although the 5-HT pathways are thought to provide a general behavioural inhibition and seem to be involved in pain suppression, sleep, thermal regulation, sexual and aggressive behaviour, as well as depression and anxiety, details of these functions are unclear. NA has a stimulating effect on the 5-HT cells.

Three classes of 5-HT receptors are recognised (5-HT-1–3).

5-HT-1A receptors include autoreceptors which inhibit 5-HT cell firing, and post-synaptic ones. Agonists include buspirone. Functional correlates include sexual behaviour and the 'serotonin syndrome' (see p. 56). 5-HT-1C receptors are widely distributed in the brain but especially in the choroid plexus and have effects on mood and appetite. 5-HT-1D receptors are found on intracranial blood vessels, where they cause vasoconstriction.

5-HT-2 receptors facilitate excitatory effects on cortical and other neurones. Ritanserin is a specific antagonist, risperidone a less specific one.

5-HT-3 receptors are pre-synaptic and activate increased release of transmitters including DA in the caudate putamen in animals. Antagonists include ondansetron which has anti-emetic effects in man (probably acting in the area postrema) and analgesic effects in animals. There are few 5-HT-3 receptors in the human brain.

The psychotomimetic drug LSD (lysergic acid diethylamide) acts on 5-HT receptors. One action is to inhibit cell firing by stimulating autoreceptors, but other actions are thought to be important in its hallucinogenic effects.

Histamine

Histamine-containing neurones exist in the hypothalamus and mid-brain reticular formation, and axons are distributed to the hypothalamus and to the forebrain. Histamine is thought to be a transmitter involved in food intake, hormonal regulation and arousal.

Three types of receptors are recognised: H-1 receptors are the site of action of classical antihistamines; H-2 receptors are also present in the brain, their function unknown, but H-2 antagonists such as cimetidine and ranitidine may cause hallucinations; H-3 receptors are autoreceptors.

GABA

GABA is a widespread inhibitory transmitter, mostly in inter-neurones in the brain. It is formed from L-glutamic acid by glutamate decarboxylase. This is a B_6-dependent enzyme, and B_6 deficiency leads to low levels of GABA and fits. Released GABA is broken down by a transaminase, but a reuptake mechanism exists to transport it back into the nerve ending.

GABA receptors are of two types. GABA-A receptors are ligand-gated channels for chloride ions. Receptor activation causes reduced excitability of the membrane. The receptor is a multi-subunit complex that can be modulated by benzodiazepines, barbiturates and steroids attaching at different sites. It is likely that there are many different GABA-receptor subtypes. Benzodiazepines interact with the receptor to potentiate the action of GABA. Benzodiazepine antagonists block this effect, for instance flumazenil. By contrast, inverse agonists decrease the effects of GABA and are anxiogenic. Barbiturates also potentiate GABA but by attaching to a different site. Picrotoxin blocks the GABA chloride channel and produces seizures. There are thought to be endogenous compounds which interact at these sites but they are not yet defined.

GABA-B receptors regulate second messengers and are also inhibitory. Baclofen is an agonist but also releases GABA.

Glutamic acid

This is an important excitatory transmitter in the brain. As yet relatively little is known of its function. Its receptors are similar to GABA-A receptors but contain a cationic channel for sodium and calcium. Phencyclidine (PCP) is thought to bind within the channel. There is a major glutamate pathway from the frontal cortex to the corpus striatum. Glutamate is implicated in learning, and in convulsive disorders.

Hormones and receptors

Hormones have important interactions with neurotransmitters and their receptors. For example, high levels of thyroid hormones lead to the up-regulation of NA beta-receptors, contributing to the features of sympathetic overactivity in thyrotoxicosis. High levels of oestrogens, as occur in pregnancy, have antipsychotic-like effects on DA receptors, and lead to up-regulation of receptor numbers; after delivery the decline in oestrogen levels leaves these receptors exposed. High levels of steroids derived from progesterone also occur in pregnancy; they have actions on GABA-A receptors similar to those of benzodiazepines.

Given these actions it is not surprising that endocrine conditions and the puerperium are associated with psychiatric disorders.

Peptides

Many peptides are thought to have roles as neurotransmitters or modulators: more than 80 have been identified. These include opioid peptides, cholecystokinin, corticotrophin releasing factor, vasointestinal peptide, neurotensin, somatostatin and angiotensin II. The most studied are the opioids because of the existence of drugs such as morphine and naltrexone which are agonist and antagonist. At least three types of receptors – mu, delta, and kappa – are recognised.

Further reading

COOPER, J.R., BLOOM, F.E. & ROTH, R.H. (1991) *The Biochemical Basis of Neuropharmacology.* Oxford: Oxford University Press.

4   Developing new drugs

The development of new drugs involves many different skills. In a pharmaceutical company, chemists synthesise new compounds by modifying existing molecules. The new compound is quickly screened for the target activity, by biochemists using test-tube techniques and by pharmacologists using *in vitro* methods and 'animal models'. If it is found to be effective, it is screened for acute toxic effects. Having passed these tests it will be studied more extensively in animals to establish its pharmacology. Toxicologists will define its safe limits before use in man and will study its disposition, metabolism and excretion. Studies of reproduction, teratology and mutagenicity will be carried out. Only after evaluation of the data for several species, and of experience with similar compounds, is the drug studied in man.

The clinical development of a new drug is divided into four phases. Each phase should be conducted by investigators with relevant expertise and facilities. Each study is based upon a detailed protocol approved by a national regulatory body and a local ethics committee, and requires informed consent by the participating individuals.

In phase 1 the basic pharmacokinetics, tolerability (side-effects), toxicity and mechanism of action are studied. Safety is the most important consideration and extreme caution is the by-word. Healthy young male volunteers free from all other drugs are generally used, because their bodies have intact homoeostatic mechanisms and are the most resilient to trauma. Single and multiple doses are studied and responses monitored. Radioactive labelling is sometimes used to assist in studying metabolism and disposition if these are complex and other assays cannot be used. These studies should reveal a safe starting dose for use in patients. Further phase 1 studies can be conducted later in other groups, for example, the elderly or physically ill.

In phase II, patients receive the drug for the first time, taking a range of doses in open studies. These cannot prove efficacy but will give pointers, and are very important for checking tolerability, and determining doses to be used in later studies. Fewer than 100 patients may be involved.

The 'pivotal studies' to prove whether the drug is effective usually require double-blind controlled trials against placebo involving 100 or so patients (late phase II trials).

Phase III contains the main therapeutic studies, to gain information about efficacy and safety in larger groups and varied settings. A few thousand patients are likely to participate, and such studies provide information about the characteristics of those who do or do not respond.

The results of these studies are submitted to the national regulatory agency to seek approval for a licence to market the drug. The time between synthesis and marketing of a new psychotropic compound is about 8–12 years. The cost of developing one new antidepressant launched in 1990 was about $300 million; in 1992 the drug earned $800 million in the USA alone.

Phase IV, the post-marketing phase, involves monitoring of the wider and more prolonged use of the drug. Different groups of patients, especially the elderly, are the subject of further controlled trials and the drug is studied in a wider range of conditions and combinations. Rarer side-effects should be detected. For instance, if a side-effect occurs in one patient in 1000, then 3000 patients will need to receive the drug in order to have a 95% probability that one patient suffers the side-effect.

This phase continues as long as the drug is on the market, and determines the drug's efficacy and safety in routine use. The occurrence of adverse drug reactions (ADRs) and the utilisation (marketing, distribution, prescribing, and use of drugs in society) are monitored. Spontaneous, voluntary reporting (the yellow-card system in Britain) and hospital-based 'intensive monitoring' are the most widely used systems for ADR assessment in this phase.

The yellow-card system is the most powerful means of first detecting new risks and has led to new psychotropic compounds being withdrawn from the market, because of haemolytic anaemia or Guillain-Barré syndrome, for example. Its usefulness depends upon the regular participation of sufficient numbers of prescribers.

ADRs should be reported if they relate to a new drug, represent previously unknown effects, or result in severe impairment or death, or neonatal malformation. Intensive monitoring includes 'case-control' studies in which patients taking the drug are compared with others who are not, but who are matched for relevant factors such as age, sex and diagnosis. Drug utilisation is studied by market research companies who persuade random samples of prescribing doctors to provide copies of their prescriptions.

Clinical trials

The design of a clinical trial involves a balance between ethical, scientific, clinical and regulatory requirements. The protocol for a trial will be submitted for approval by the regulatory authority (Department of Health) who must issue a certificate if it is to proceed. The protocol is then submitted by the investigator to the local ethics committee.

Many studies are based on the randomly assigned, double-blind, parallel group, comparative design, using a placebo or active control, or both. This powerful design was conceived by Bradford Hill during World War II and kept secret as part of the British war effort. Sometimes, especially for rarer conditions, within-patient designs are used, in which the same patient is studied on different treatments, as in the placebo crossover study or Latin square design. Cessation studies are important for studying rebound phenomena and withdrawal syndromes, and for assessing prophylactic efficacy.

Ethics

Ethical principles provide guidance as to what ought to be done and what can be done, and are particularly complex in psychiatry where the ability of the person to make decisions is affected by mental illness. Respect for individuals' rights and their desire to contribute to research is balanced by the collective need to develop optimal treatments, and by common sense. Development of better treatment and knowledge of which treatment is best can only be achieved by systematic medical experimentation involving patients.

The Helsinki Declarations (1964 and 1975) provide a framework for ethical clinical research, adapted by the World Health Organization. These and local laws and codes govern the planning of clinical trials. Their application to a specific project is assessed by a group of people knowledgeable about local ethical, cultural, medical and legal issues (ethics committee). The committee should review the research protocol for the questions of informed consent of the subject, the balance of risks and expected benefits, and confidentiality. They should also ensure that proper insurance exists in the event of damage to the individual, arising from adherence to the protocol, or negligence of the staff.

Participation in a trial is voluntary. Consent is given and witnessed after the patient has received adequate and accurate information including a standard form of words, written in a clear way that they can understand. They should be free to withdraw from the study at any time, and if they do not wish to participate they should still be able to receive the usual treatment for their condition.

Placebo

To prove efficacy in psychiatric conditions, it is necessary to design studies that take account of spontaneous improvement, and of bias in the observer or patient. This can be achieved by having a control group, assigning patients at random to receive either the new treatment or a comparator, and conducting the trial double-blind (neither the doctor nor the patient knowing which treatment is received until all the data from the whole trial are gathered and complete). If a new treatment is much better than the standard treatment, then only these two groups are needed. If, however, the new drug is thought to be about as effective as standard treatment, and if the condition is liable to spontaneous improvement, then efficacy can only be proved by comparison with placebo. Regulatory authorities in many countries require two 'pivotal studies' in separate centres to show superiority to placebo, before a drug can be licensed for use in a psychiatric condition. It is best to include both placebo and standard treatment as comparators since this will show whether the standard treatment is effective under the circumstances of the trial; if not, the trial fails as a test of efficacy.

The inclusion of placebo in a study will mean that patients cannot be included if they require immediate active treatment, for example because they are severely disturbed.

In deciding whether to ask an individual patient to participate in a study, the investigator must balance the needs of the study with those of the patient.

Trial protocol

This should describe the rationale for the study. The selection of patients should be based on inclusion and exclusion criteria; the relevant diagnosis is reached according to standard criteria (such as the World Health Organization's ICD–10 or the American Psychiatric Association's DSM–IV) and a particular level of severity on a standard rating scale. The age range, sex, and race of the patients may be specified. Exclusion criteria should include females who are at risk of pregnancy, patients with somatic illnesses, and those who are taking certain other medication or have a history of alcohol or drug abuse. The number of patients to be recruited to the study should be determined in advance, based upon advice from a statistician. The number should be sufficient to avoid the possibility of a type II statistical error (false-negative result). The patients may be subdivided or 'stratified', for instance according to the number and pattern of previous episodes, and assigned randomly to receive one of the study treatments. The dosage may be variable, fixed, or variable within pre-set limits.

The use of more than one dose range of active treatment allows dose-response relations to be explored, and compared with the incidence of side-effects. There should be a wash-out period before entry to the study to avoid interactions with previous medication, and to identify patients who improve spontaneously and are therefore best not included. During the trial, additional medication should be avoided as far as possible. Medication such as night sedation or anti-cholinergic drugs should be standardised.

The patient should be assessed regularly, using validated clinical rating scales for their condition. The scales should be comprehensive, sensitive to change, and easy to apply in the circumstances of the trial. In multi-centre studies it is important to hold training sessions to improve inter-rater reliability, as this improves the power of the study. Global assessments and self-reports of improvement should also be recorded. Side-effects can be measured by standard checklists and by open enquiry. Laboratory tests are monitored at relevant intervals as part of routine safety checks. Blood levels of the drug are measured both to confirm adherence to treatment and to explore the relationship between blood level and efficacy.

All the data should be collected before the trial code is broken, showing which patient received which treatment. The results should be analysed using appropriate statistical methods, preferably by a statistician independent of the investigators. Patients who drop out or who are withdrawn through side-effects, non-response or recovery, pose difficulties for the analysis. When studying the results of a trial it is important to know whether the scores from these drop-outs have been included in subsequent analyses ('last value carried forward') or only to the time of drop out ('intention to treat analysis').

The information gathered during the trial must respect the patient's confidentiality and must be preserved for several years. Pharmaceutical companies are expected to monitor trials to ensure that they are conducted according to national requirements for good clinical practice, including the external audit of case notes and of the trial record-books.

The results of well conducted clinical trials should be published, even if the results are unfavourable to the new drug.

Further reading

DOLL, R. (1990) The development of controlled trials in preventative and therapeutic medicine. *Journal of Biosocial Science*, **23**, 365–378.

GROF, P., AKHTER, M.T., CAMPBELL, M., *et al* (1993) *Clinical Evaluation of Psychotropic Drugs for Psychiatric Disorders*. WHO Expert Series on Biological Psychiatry, Vol. 2. Seattle: Hogrefe & Huber.

ROYAL COLLEGE OF PSYCHIATRISTS (1990) Guidelines for research ethics committees on psychiatric research involving human subjects. *Psychiatric Bulletin*, **14**, 48–61.

5 Clinical practice

The fact that a drug has been prescribed is no guarantee that the patient has actually fetched the tablets from a pharmacy, or taken them in the number and the frequency instructed. In hospital, nurses sometimes withhold doses. Mistakes in administration of drugs occur, patients getting too much, too little or someone else's prescription. Furthermore, some patients who seem to accept the prescribed treatment may secretly palm and throw away their tablets, or hide them in their mouths and secretly spit them out. This is why liquid preparations may be more effective than tablets, and injections surer still.

Whenever a drug seems to fail or to produce unusual results, it is wise to check that it has in fact been taken as instructed. Look at the tablet bottle, ask the patient and the nurse directly, remember that urine tests or blood level measurements exist for some drugs.

Complaints of side-effects result at least as often for psychological as they do for pharmacological reasons. That is often the reason when the patient is upset after only one or two doses, and especially when the dose is small.

True physical sensitivities are rare, psychological sensitivities common. Psychological sensitivities may take the form of anxiety, preoccupation with bodily perceptions, mistrust of doctor or nurse, exaggerated ideas about 'drugs' and their risks, for instance poisoning, addiction, loss of self-control. The doctor must be alive to the patient's attitude to his own body, to his mistrust, to his view of tablets and medicines, if necessary bringing his feelings into open discussion, and possibly modifying the treatment plan if feelings are strong. Confidence is created by giving the patients time, showing concern for them and asking about their family and work situation in relation to their illness. It means being unhurried, calm, sincere and confident. The patient who has confidence in the doctor will tolerate the experience of many side-effects without complaint and they may be discovered only on direct enquiry.

It is usually helpful to explain to patients in simple language what each drug is supposed to do for them and the logic of its use, and to add something about the more common side-effects and what they mean. How this is done must be suited to the intelligence and previous knowledge of the individual patient, and take into account obsessional or hypochondriacal tendencies. For some drugs, lithium in particular, the pharmacist gives a leaflet with advice on side-effects, interactions, and signs of toxicity. More intense education is useful for relatives and patients undergoing long-term treatment for a severe illness.

On the positive side, the patient's confidence, suggestibility, belief in the potency of a remedy – which may depend in part on its striking colour or bitter taste – acceptance of the doctor's 'gift' of tablets as symbolic or magical, involving concern or care, the prestige of medical knowledge, and so on, just as much as pharmacology, are factors in the acceptability of treatment. Patients may complain of side-effects, or indeed get better, when treated with tablets without any active drug within them. This placebo effect may add to the pharmacological effect where an active drug is also used. The overall effectiveness of treatment, therefore, depends very much on creating the right psychological conditions as well as prescribing the right drug in the right dose.

Two of the most common reasons for poor results in drug treatment are inadequate dosage, and failure to go on long enough. Frequent newspaper criticism of overprescribing, or of turning people into zombies, persuades doctors to prescribe too little. Some patients try to control their own treatment and demand changes of dose or drug. The doctor should be the technical expert here, with enough clinical knowledge not to be diverted from assessment of the seriousness of the illness, and the pharmacological measures it requires. If a high dose is given too soon, intolerable side-effects may occur before the drug has time to produce beneficial effects.

Points to remember

Work with a few established drugs and know them well

Begin by knowing the use of a few drugs thoroughly rather than a large list superficially. Start with drugs whose dose range, side-effects, contraindications and interactions are known from extensive use in clinical practice. Only use newly launched drugs of limited experience if they have some clear advantage.

Avoid prescribing more than one drug of the same chemical class at the same time

There is usually no clinical advantage in giving, say, amitriptyline with imipramine, or chlorpromazine with thioridazine. Treatment is complicated needlessly, and patient and nurse burdened unnecessarily with extra tablets. Increase a dose, rather than add a second drug for fear of exceeding some recommended maximum of the first.

Identify appropriate target symptoms

Be sure that the symptom targeted to monitor improvement is part of the illness, rather than the personality. Sleep and appetite often improve in depression before other symptoms do.

If a drug fails, change to one of a different chemical group

When a drug fails, change to a drug from a different group. If an adequate dose of amitriptyline does not relieve depression, try an SSRI or an MAOI rather than another tricyclic.

Change one thing at a time

Only by doing this can one learn whether a particular treatment is effective or ineffective.

Prescribing 'as required' (p.r.n.) can be risky

Prescribing 'as required' is potentially dangerous because staff who may not have the appropriate clinical or pharmacological knowledge are authorised to give unlimited extra doses of potentially toxic and interacting drugs.

The best practice for discretionary medication is written instructions limiting the number of repetitions and their duration, for example, "Repeat dose once, if needed, any night in the next five", or specify the maximum dose in 24 hours.

Do not prescribe more than three psychotropic drugs at once

Every symptom does not have to be treated; attempting to do so results in excessive prescribing.

A large number of medicines is a burden to patient, relative or nurse. Errors of dose and timing are more likely to occur, and disrupt the regular timetable of medication. More drugs increase the chance of drug interactions.

Hypnotics may not be necessary to control insomnia

The prescription of an hypnotic to control sleeplessness can be avoided by giving sedative tricyclics and phenothiazines.

Time tablet-taking to suit the patient's lifestyle

Prescribing a drug to be taken three times a day can become an unthinking habit. Perhaps the drug can be given once a day at a convenient and easily remembered time such as going to bed. Dose-related side-effects are more likely with the midday dose because it is so close to the early morning dose. Lunch-time medication tends to be omitted by people at work who forget in the press of the day's events or are embarrassed taking tablets in public. People who work unusual hours may need advice about timing. Those who insist on drinking alcohol will need advice about when to take their drugs.

Do not reject drugs too soon as ineffective

Prescribe a big enough dose for long enough to be sure a drug has failed before stopping. Dose response cannot be predicted accurately but it can be found from trial and observation. The discovery of an effective drug and its optimal dose is of such tremendous importance to a patient with a lifetime of chronic or recurring illness that months of careful trial of drugs is worthwhile.

Women may become pregnant

Psychotropic drugs may harm the developing foetus. Before prescribing inquire about the last menstrual period and the patient's intentions about getting pregnant.

The pregnant

A depressive illness or an attack of schizophrenia during pregnancy can be devastating for the mother and potentially a serious threat to the well-being and sometimes life of the unborn child. Where there is a serious risk of a mental breakdown, the prophylactic use of a tricyclic antidepressant, or of a phenothiazine may become necessary. Psychotropic drugs may increase the risk of congenital deformities in the baby. Such abnormalities occur in at least 1–2% of pregnancies anyway, with no known cause. Animal experiments with drugs sometimes suggest teratogenicity, but because the experiments are not on humans, and usually with high doses of drugs, such suggestions have to be regarded with reserve. Only human experience of the drug, with careful collection of statistics over a long period, can be the true guide.

However, it is fair to say that if the commonly used psychotropic drugs increase the risk of damage to the foetus, most do not do so to a great extent, on present knowledge. The risk must be balanced against the consequences of serious mental illness to the mother and her family. Remember that a drug is likely to be more of a risk for the foetus in higher dosage, and during the first three months of foetal life. New drugs or those with known risks, such as carbamazepine, should be avoided.

As drug metabolism may be altered during pregnancy, adjust dosage in the pregnant, and readjust in the puerperium.

Infants

Most drugs cross the placental barrier, and also appear in breast milk. The neonate may show withdrawal symptoms if its mother is dependent on opiates or alcohol. The infant may be limp or even goitrous if the mother takes lithium, but these effects are temporary and cause no lasting harm. Even though the amounts of drug in milk may not be great, the neonate up to about one year old has less than a child or adult in the way of liver hydroxylating enzymes to destroy active drugs, and poor renal function as well. Drugs tend to persist in its body. On present knowledge the doses of phenothiazines, tricyclic antidepressants, anticonvulsants and hypnotics administered to babies in the breast milk of mothers on these drugs are unimportant. Where the mother is taking doses of lithium or diazepam, however, the baby may be affected, and therefore breast feeding is better avoided.

The elderly

As people age they enter a new phase of medical management. Growing old means metabolic impairment, often aggravated by chronic disease. Kidneys no longer excrete so well, livers no longer metabolise so fast. Small doses of drugs consequently last longer, accumulate more, and exert bigger effects. The ageing brain becomes more sensitive to some drugs, benzodiazepines and anti-Parkinsonian drugs especially.

These changes occur at different ages for different people and at different rates for different drugs, but are particularly marked in the very old. Older people may have multiple diseases and multiple prescribing, often from two or more sources. They have, therefore. a much greater tendency to toxic reactions, accidental overdosing, and drug interactions than the young. Dietary indiscretions, constipation, and inactivity may also have excessive effects on older people's well-being.

Ageing also means psychological impairment. Impaired memory and concentration cause instructions about drugs to be forgotten or muddled. If in charge of their own medication the treatment plan must be simple: few drugs, preferably no more than three, taken on a regular, easily remembered schedule, linked to the fixed points of the day – at meals or when going to bed for instance. Out-patients need written instructions – which medicines to

take and when to take them. As a check, have them bring
back unused medication from previous prescriptions. A
relative, friend, community nurse, or warden may be able
to take some responsibility for giving the drugs when there
is doubt about competence. A drug wallet may be loaded
by the pharmacist, with each day's tablets grouped into
compartments, for a whole week. Complications may arise
from self-medication with analgesics, aperients, drugs from
the last illness or even from someone else. Psychiatric
disorder in the elderly person, especially acute brain
syndrome, often results from taking too much prescribed
and non-prescribed medication.

Insomnia with a request for hypnotics is such a common
problem in the care of the elderly that a special comment
is required. Find out if the complaint can be treated by
simple measures before prescribing an hypnotic. Some
lonely old people go to bed in the early evening and get
five or six hours' sleep before their 'insomnia' begins; an
after-lunch nap may be prolonged to 6 p.m. So find out
the hours they spend in bed asleep, or trying to sleep, and
get independent confirmation.

Reading, less time in bed, or taking part in interesting
things which require some activity, may give better sleep.
Rising at a regular time helps to set circadian rhythms
including the sleep/wake cycle. Improved bedroom
comfort such as quiet, correct temperature, and pillows at
the right height, all help to promote sleep.

Sometimes diet is the culprit. Too much coffee causes
excessive arousal by bed-time. Alcohol taken in the early
evening may wear off in the night. Too much fluid during
the day can result in repeated waking with a full bladder.
Too much food of the wrong kind causes indigestion.
Constipation can lead to restlessness. Too much smoking
may impair sleep. Medical problems interfere with sleep.
Proper attention to pain, breathlessness, coughing, and
frequency and the correct timing of diuretic tablets may
result in improved sleep.

An occasional dose of a hypnotic may be used, but look
out for unwanted effects. Be prepared to try several

different preparations and aim for an early trial without hypnotics again, because the need for them may vary over time and with changing circumstances. Long-term use is generally ineffective and produces dependence. Chloral hydrate preparations and promazine may be given in doses about half the size for a younger adult. A short-acting benzodiazepine, such as temazepam, produces less hangover. Avoid barbiturates and long periods of benzodiazepines. However, for patients who have taken barbiturates or benzodiazepines for a very long time without increasing doses, the sensible and humane course may be to continue the prescription, but try to wean them from it very slowly. The alternative will be an unhappy patient and possibly withdrawal fits or a psychosis.

Excessive night sedation is dangerous. It causes mental dulling, mental confusion, incontinence, restlessness, wandering, especially at night but sometimes by day, and impairment of balance with a risk of falling. Chest infections are more likely in the heavily sedated.

Unexpected results

No effect

Failure to show any response may be due to 'non-adherence' or 'non-compliance'. The patient has simply not taken the tablets, or taken them irregularly or in less than the prescribed dose. Many patients will admit this on direct kindly questioning, or their relatives will. Otherwise a short period of in-patient nursing observation may be needed to be sure. Plasma level measurements, if available, may help. Of course, the prescribed dose may have been too little, or even too much, or the illness is truly not susceptible to the drug. But there must be sound evidence that the patient has taken the drug before such an important conclusion is reached.

New symptoms

New mental or physical symptoms other than usual side-effects may appear, particularly after 48 hours, or at around 10 days, or late in the course of chronic treatment. The important question is to decide if the symptoms result from idiosyncrasy, that is, some individual variation of metabolism or unusual immunological response (allergy). If it is, continuing the drug may be dangerous, and it may be impossible ever to give it again. It can be a serious matter if a patient with recurrent depressions or a schizophrenic illness cannot have the clinical benefits of an antidepressant or an antipsychotic because of the risks of idiosyncratic response. Therefore, it is important to collect satisfactory evidence before condemning a drug.

Unexpected results have many possible causes. The symptoms may be those of toxic overdosage, taken by mistake or design, or resulting from a dispensing or nursing error. Alternatively, the patient may be intolerant of a usually safe dose of the drug because of an inability to metabolise it normally. That may happen because of an individual metabolic difference, or because some other drug taken at the same time interferes with normal metabolism. Attention to the dose or to the other drugs, may put matters right. There may be a coincident onset of a physical illness, which makes the patient intolerant of his usual dose, or produces symptoms such as vomiting or diarrhoea which are mistaken for a toxic reaction.

The idiosyncrasy may not be due to the drug you have prescribed but to some other drug the patient has taken, or even to food. For example, bronchospasm can result from aspirin sensitivity; urticarial rash and fever can be produced by crabmeat. Remember that an allergic idiosyncrasy is sometimes to the coating of a tablet, or to the excipient or vehicle, for instance the oil of a depot injection, and not to the active drug itself. The idiosyncrasy may be due to a toxic metabolite, for example agranulocytosis with chlorpromazine, or may be allergic, such as cholestatic jaundice, also with chlorpromazine.

The symptoms of idiosyncrasy may be:

(a)   in the skin: purpura, urticaria, maculopapular rash, exfoliative dermatitis
(b)   in the lung: bronchospasm
(c)   in the kidney: albuminuria, haemoglobinuria, signs of oliguria and nephritis
(d)   in the liver: jaundice
(e)   in the blood: sudden drop in platelets, red cell or white cell count (agranulocytosis) (this may present with fever, sore throat or rash)
(f)   a sudden rise in temperature, with joint pains, swollen glands, and urticaria, 8–10 days after starting may be due to serum sickness, from excess drug antigen reacting with antibody
(g)   Stevens-Johnson syndrome: a severe multi-organ inflammatory reaction with skin and mucosal lesions and pneumonia
(h)   a neuroleptic malignant syndrome (see p. 56).

What to do in case of suspected idiosyncrasy

Stop the suspected drug: stop all drugs if that is feasible. Take 10 ml blood and deep-freeze the serum for possible later immunological study. Take a careful drug and chemical history, not only what a doctor has prescribed but what nurses have given or the patient taken of his own accord, for instance proprietary medicines, and what foods, drinks, or industrial chemicals the patient has encountered.

The advice and help of physician, dermatologist and clinical pathologist should be sought. Treatment with corticosteroids may be needed to help the patient over the damage. Blood and urine tests may be needed. Skin tests (prick and scratch or patch) may be advisable to confirm the existence of hypersensitivity.

There may be a possibility of desensitisation. Idiosyncrasy established to one antipsychotic, for instance, does not ban all. If the patient's psychiatric state requires drug treatment, start cautiously with another drug, small doses at first, slowly increasing, with daily monitoring of skin and temperature and twice-weekly blood counts and urine analyses until four weeks have passed.

Do not forget to report this drug reaction to the Committee on Safety of Medicines, Freepost, London SW8 5BR.

If it is safe to do so, the link between the drug and the idiosyncrasy may be proved by re-exposure in a double-blind way, with placebo.

In some instances of hepatic sensitivity, the drug can be given again later without the problem recurring, but the advice of a specialist physician must be sought.

Look out for these

Unusual reactions can be idiosyncratic, due to an individual's metabolic abnormality or organic pathology, or an acquired allergy. But many are simply rarely observed side-effects, caused perhaps by an over-rapid rise to high drug dose in treatment, or by an over-rapid drug withdrawal, outpacing the central nervous system's capacity to adapt biochemically. Others are the signs of interaction with another drug in the therapy.

However, some reports of unusual reactions are mistaken: the reactions are not due to a psychotropic drug at all but to a missed organic illness, or to some other chemical with which the patient is in contact, possibly self-prescribed. This is why unusual reactions should be investigated pathologically, in the fullest possible way (including a post-mortem if the patient has died), instead of jumping to some guessed conclusion.

In its early days, chlorpromazine was frequently thought to damage the liver, but later study showed there had been coincident infective hepatitis; also, the simple test for bile pigments in urine, used to detect occult liver damage, was made positive by metabolites of chlorpromazine alone.

Although many reactions are described in their place elsewhere in this book, it may be helpful to list some reactions that are not always considered, but are important.

Rapid rise to high dose

(a) Bizarre movements of tongue, back, or limbs, thought to be attention-seeking ('hysterical') or neurological disease, are due to neuroleptic-induced dystonia (see p. 135).
(b) Nausea, dizziness or drowsiness with antidepressants.
(c) Ataxia, clumsiness, slurred speech and vomiting due to high lithium levels.

Rapid withdrawal after long-term treatment

(a) Delirium tremens, from alcohol.
(b) Epileptic fit, from benzodiazepine or barbiturate.
(c) Manic attack, two to four weeks after stopping lithium.
(d) Headache, nausea, vomiting, insomnia, from imipramine or amitriptyline, or a phenothiazine.
(e) Severe Parkinsonism, with rigidity, salivation, from loss of anti-Parkinsonian drug.
(f) Sudden reduction of high dose may result in confusional state.
(g) Dizziness after SSRIs, for example paroxetine.
(h) Nausea, feeling of unsteadiness as if on a boat, and visual illusions after benzodiazepines.

Drug interaction

(a) Severe throbbing headache with hypertension and sometimes fever from MAOI, with amine drug such as tricyclic, or ephedrine (in cold cure).

  (b) Parkinsonism from tricyclic plus lithium.
  (c) 'Serotonin syndrome': high fever, myoclonus,
       confusion, fits and coma, from combination of
       drugs increasing serotonin function, for example
       SSRIs with MAOIs, lithium, L-tryptophan, or
       carbamazepine.
  (d) Lithium toxicity at relatively low blood levels,
       especially in combination with antipsychotics or
       other drugs.

Neuroleptic malignant syndrome

This consists of generalised muscular rigidity (which can
make swallowing and breathing difficult), pyrexia, autonomic
instability, and lowered consciousness. Laboratory findings
include raised creatine phosphokinase (CPK), leucocytosis,
and low serum iron. It occurs during treatment with
antipsychotics and is thought to be due to diminished
dopamine function in the basal ganglia and possibly the
hypothalamus. Its cause is unclear but antipsychotics must
be stopped or the outcome may be fatal with hyperpyrexia
and pneumonia. It is more likely to occur during an
intercurrent physical illness, or in a patient with catatonic
features. A detailed physical examination and investigations
should be made. After full recovery, the patient may be
able to tolerate the same drug again without a recurrence,
but it is best if possible to use drugs of a different class.
All classes of antipsychotics can cause it. For severe cases,
treatment may be tried with bromocriptine (5–60 mg, daily)
or with dantrolene which acts directly on skeletal muscle;
the advice of a specialist physician should be sought, urgently.

Unexpected Parkinsonism

Do not forget that haloperidol, even when given for only
a short period, can provoke this reaction, which may then
continue for up to six months after the drug has been

stopped. Also, a patient who develops a depressive illness may show some signs of Parkinsonism, which will disappear again as the patient recovers. (See also akathisia, p. 135, and tardive dyskinesia, p. 136.)

6   Good prescribing habits

In-patients

The prescription sheet serves four separate but interrelated functions. It is the means of ordering drugs from the pharmacy, it is the instruction sheet for nurses giving patients the drug, it records the administration, and it is also an important part of the patient's record of treatment. It may also become a legal document in litigation. Different hospitals have different designs of treatment chart. The following procedures are worth putting into practice.

(a)   The patient's surname, first name, date of birth, hospital number and ward should always be on the prescription sheet. Do not leave it to someone else.

(b)   Date the prescription.

(c)   Use the proper name of the drug, not its commercial term, unless a particular brand is intended. State the form in which the drug is to be given.

(d)   Write, preferably print, in English when the drug is to be given and do not use medical Latin, or abbreviations such as 'b.d.' or 'p.r.n.' which result in error.

(e)   In writing 'as required' medication, give maximum dosage at any one time, possible dose frequency, and total dosage within 24 hours. For use in acute disturbance, limit the number of days it is valid, for example seven. Do not write 'oral/i.m.', but write separate prescriptions for each route, or it will later be impossible to tell which route was used, and smaller doses are needed intramuscularly.

(f) Sign the prescription legibly with name as well as initials.

(g) At the same time as you prescribe a drug, write in the case notes what you have prescribed and give a reason, assessing the effects of the previous drug if there was one.

(h) When changing a prescription, date the crossing-out of the previous drug when the new drug is written in.

(i) In long-term patients review medication at least monthly; in acute cases, at least weekly. Check from time to time how the nurses are giving out a prescription. For instance, night sedation may be given routinely needlessly, or too early, or daytime sedation may be overused.

(j) File old prescription cards in sequence so that it is a simple matter to find out what medication the patient had been receiving at an earlier date.

Out-patients

The hospital pharmacy may supply drugs for out-patients, usually on a special hospital card; otherwise drugs for out-patient treatment in the National Health Service (NHS) may be prescribed on form FP10(HP), pads of which are provided by the hospital. An FP10 form is, in effect, an order to a commercial pharmacist to supply the drugs written on it to the patient whose name appears at the top, in return for payment, part of which is met by the patient and the remainder by the NHS.

The FP10 form is also a set of instructions to the pharmacist about what to write on the label so that patients may know what they are taking, how often to take it and for how long. The FP10 may become a legal document in cases of litigation. Since the FP10 form cannot be a record of treatment unless carbon copies are kept, a note of the prescription should also be made in the patient's case notes, dated and signed. Remember to observe the following.

With the patient's full name and address at the top, print the proper name of the drug, not its commercial name unless you intend a particular brand to be dispensed. Specify the form in which it is to be dispensed, the frequency in which it is to be taken, and the number of tablets, capsules, and so on which are to be given to the patient. The pharmacist must supply what is written – standard preparation or particular commercial brand – except in the case of Government-approved 'listed' drugs, mainly benzodiazepines, for which a generic brand may be dispensed even when, for instance, Valium is written. (See Chapter 7.)

If you do not wish your patient to know the drug name, delete the letters 'NP' at the top of the prescription form, otherwise the dispenser will write the name of the drug on the container label. Sign and print your name legibly; if there is a mistake the dispenser will be able to contact you.

Explain to patients why the drug is given and tell them, or a responsible relative, how often to take it, what serious side-effects to expect, and how to cope with them. Failure to take drugs results in part from poor instruction.

Since the FP10 is in the patient's charge between leaving the out-patient clinic and reaching the dispensing chemist, opportunity for forgery arises. To avoid forgery, print the drug name in bold capitals and the quantity in arabic numerals and in words. Leave no free space below the prescription and initial alterations.

Prescriptions ordering controlled drugs are covered by certain restrictions (see p. 177). Remember, FP10 pads can be stolen and used to forge prescriptions. Lock them up.

One principle governing the role of the hospital or general practitioner (GP) in prescribing is that the doctor who has clinical responsibility for that element of a patient's care should do the prescribing. The high cost of new medicines and the fact that hospital doctors may prescribe drugs to treat conditions with which the GP is less familiar have led to the need for 'shared care' for some conditions. This is most appropriate for the long-term management of chronic but stabilised illness, such as bipolar affective disorder. For these conditions the hospital doctor and the GP must agree on a written arrangement – protocol – setting out who does what, for instance the arrangements for prescribing, blood tests, and medical review. This is also suitable for other conditions, such as prescribing for schizophrenics or for addicts.

Dependence on prescribed drugs

Usually anxiety, tension, worrying, and helplessness first bring these patients to medical attention. They want regular doses of minor tranquillisers, analgesics, or appetite suppressants to avert symptoms and to maintain a sense of well-being, but they do not become dependent on hard drugs. By the time they reach psychiatric out-patient care, they have usually been provided with drugs for years. Referral may be by GPs no longer agreeable to prescribe such drugs long-term, or by patients themselves, influenced by the media emphasising the dangers, wishing to withdraw.

Psychiatrists may decide to advise continuing the supply of drugs but they must take steps to ensure that drug intake does not steadily increase, as it may easily do, by agreeing with the family doctor for only one person to prescribe the drug and to fix what the dose shall be. On the other hand, if the agreed aim is withdrawal, appropriate psychological help, usually by group method, is needed. Whichever course is decided, the longer-term management is a matter for the family doctor.

Further reading

BARRETT, C.W. & TOMES, J. (1992) Shared care – the way forward. *Hospital Update Plus*, April, 7–10.

7   The cost of treatment

To the National Health Service

The prescriber should have some idea of the price of drugs and, hence, the cost of a course of treatment in the short and long term, so as to make the best use of National Health Service (NHS) money. Even in non-inflationary times, drug prices change. A drug is usually expensive when new and cheaper later, when generic equivalents become available on the expiry of patents. Even so, the more expensive branded preparation may, under certain circumstances, be preferable to the generic product, easier to swallow, more palatable, possess a longer shelf-life after manufacture, or have superior bioavailability.

The approximate cost to the NHS of branded drugs can be obtained from the *Monthly Index of Medical Specialities* (MIMS), or from the six-monthly *British National Formulary* (BNF). MIMS provides, as a guide to prescribing in practice, a classified list of drugs which may be prescribed or recommended including, for most drugs, the retail price. The BNF also lists prices which are, whenever possible, based on basic net prices. The cost of dispensing a prescription from a retail pharmacy includes the professional fees and overheads which are not included in MIMS or BNF prices. Hospital pharmacy prices are often much lower than those of retail pharmacists because a local or national bulk purchasing contract has been arranged with the supplier. The hospital pharmacist will know this. To illustrate variable costs, the purchase prices for commonly prescribed psychotropic drugs cited in BNF (March 1993) are compared with hospital contract prices from one district (NHS Trust) (Table 1).

Districts vary widely in what they have been able to negotiate in buying a particular brand of drug, especially if they purchase very large amounts. In the example given, the particular district had negotiated a reduced price for 'Priadel' but not for 'Camcolit' (see Table 1). Hospital prices include VAT; MIMS prices are exclusive of VAT, as are those in the BNF.

TABLE 1

Comparison of drug costs to the NHS: retail (BNF) prices and hospital contract prices (including VAT) (March 1993)

Drugs	Hospital purchase: £	BNF: £ + VAT
Tricyclics: 75 mg a day for 28 days (84 x 25 mg tablets)		
Imipramine	0.46	0.59
'Tofranil'	—	3.11
Clomipramine	6.38	6.38
'Anafranil'	6.38	6.38
Amitriptyline	0.38	0.40
'Tryptizol'	—	2.27
'Lentizol'	—	4.55
Newer antidepressants: for 28 days		
Lofepramine: 210 mg daily ('Gamanil', 70 mg tablet)	14.32	17.57
Fluvoxamine: 150 mg daily ('Faverin', 50 mg tablet)	23.03	40.12
Fluoxetine: 20 mg daily ('Prozac', 20 mg tablet)	9.13	25.11
Moclobemide: 300 mg daily ('Manerix', 150 mg tablet)	23.03	23.03
Paroxetine: 20 mg daily ('Seroxat', 20 mg tablet)	13.39	37.18
Sertraline: 100 mg daily ('Lustral', 100 mg tablet)	—	46.73
Trazodone: 300 mg daily ('Molipaxin', 150 mg tablet)	—	27.31

TABLE 1 (continued)

Drugs	Hospital purchase: £	BNF: £ + VAT
Lithium: (1600 mg a day for 25 days)		
'Camcolit': 400 mg	3.81	3.81
'Priadel': 400 mg	1.44	3.64
Antipsychotics: (12 days' treatment)		
Chlorpromazine: 400 mg daily (100 mg tablet)	1.01	2.17
'Largactil': 400 mg (100 mg tablet)	—	2.17
Thioridazine: 400 mg (100 mg tablet)	2.55	3.10
'Melleril': 400 mg (100 mg tablet)	—	3.27
Haloperidol: 30 mg daily (10 mg tablet)	1.21	—
'Haldol': 30 mg daily (10 mg tablet)	—	6.98
Syrup		
Chlorpromazine 25 mg/5 ml (500 ml)	1.90	3.47
'Largactil' 25 mg/5 ml (500 ml)	—	3.47
Thioridazine 25 mg/5 ml (500 ml)	1.90	—
'Melleril' 25 mg/5 ml (500 ml)	—	4.58
Non-sedative and atypical antipsychotics: (for 28 days)		
Pimozide ('Orap', 4 mg tablet)	36.23	41.39
Sulpiride: 800 mg daily ('Dolmatil', 200 mg tablet)	15.20	27.64
Trifluoperazine: 20 mg daily ('Stelazine', spansule 10 mg)	3.88	3.88
Remoxipride: 300 mg daily ('Roxiam', 300 mg tablet)	—	25.33
Risperidone: 6 mg daily ('Risperdal', 3 mg tablet)	—	131.60
Clozapine: 300 mg daily ('Clozaril', 100 mg tablet)	163.00	181.00

Syrup takes more time to give than tablets because nursing staff have to measure the dose. However, it is more difficult to disguise not taking syrup. Syrup is more expensive than tablets dose for dose, and injections are dearer still.

It is important to know the expensive drugs and prescribe them for a good reason. 'Anafranil' or clomipramine compared with 'Tryptizol' or amitriptyline is an example. But cost can be overemphasised as a factor in clinical decisions. Psychotropic drugs are inexpensive compared with drugs used in general medicine. Concentrate on choosing the right drug without getting distracted by the difference between 3p and 5p a day.

The very high cost of giving clozapine to 'treatment-resistant' schizophrenic patients is on a different level. In economic terms, studies have suggested that the better functioning and increased longevity of a responsive patient offsets the drug's high cost. But, on ethical grounds, it would seem right to give a drug, however expensive and if safe, to a patient crippled by illness. Likewise, the cost of new antidepressants is balanced by their greater safety in overdose.

To the patient

All prescriptions written on FP10 forms cost the patient £4.25 (April 1993 price) for each drug, each time it is dispensed. These charges can be a sizeable financial burden for patients requiring multiple drugs long term, especially if poor as so many continuing care patients are. However, prescription charges can be mitigated. The NHS has ruled that prescriptions for some medical conditions are exempt from charges. Patients with these conditions do not have to pay charges for their psychotropic drugs. This applies, for instance, to epilepsy, diabetes, hypothyroidism and thyrotoxicosis. There are other exceptions. The following groups are exempt from prescription charges: children under 16, those in full-time education (up to 19 years), women over 60, men over 65, pregnant women, women with children under one year, and people receiving income support, family credit, war or service disablement pensions if the treatment is of a condition caused by a disablement.

Prescription charges for patients who have to pay can be reduced with a 'season ticket' which costs £22.00 for four months and £60.60 for twelve months. These are worthwhile for more than five prescribed items or repeats in four months and 14 over a year. 'Season tickets' can be obtained by applying on form FP95/EC95, available from post offices, social security offices, family practitioner committees or retail pharmacists.

Limited prescribing

In April 1986 the Department of Health and Social Security, to reduce the cost of medicines to the NHS, introduced limited prescribing for five categories of medicines. This arose because of arbitrary prescribing of pharmacologically similar preparations of widely varying price. One category deals with tranquillisers and sedatives. As a result, general practitioners can only prescribe, using their generic name, those tranquillisers and sedatives on the approved list. Drugs not prescribable under the NHS are identified in MIMS and the BNF by a symbol. Non-approved drugs can still be prescribed on private prescriptions.

Hospitals are not obliged to follow this restriction and, in many instances, hospital doctors can still prescribe a wider range of psychotropic drugs from their hospital pharmacies than can general practitioners. However, hospital doctors must observe the restrictions if they write prescriptions on FP10(HP) forms for retail pharmacists. Many hospitals have, through consultation between clinicians and pharmacists, developed guidelines for prescribing embodying the principles of the limited list. These district drug formularies, which give information on uses, dosage and costs of selected drugs, have an important role to play in reducing the cost of medicines without sacrificing quality of treatment.

Part II. Approaches to treatment

8 Depressive illness

Depression is the name of a feeling and is usually but not always accompanied by a sad face, tears, or complaints of gloom and pessimism. The doctor is only called in when the feeling seems inappropriate in strength, duration, or occasion. To feel depressed for a few hours now and then is normal, but to be depressed for days, weeks or months on end is quite another matter. This inappropriate depression may be a primary part of the symptom complex of a depressive illness, or a secondary consequence of some other illness or disability. Discrimination between these possibilities affects the treatment.

Pathophysiology

Depressive illness is a common condition affecting about 3% of the population in a severe form in any six-month period, and it tends to recur. Biochemical theories about the underlying pathophysiology are based largely upon the effects of drugs. Thus drugs such as reserpine, which deplete the biogenic amines noradrenaline, serotonin and dopamine, can cause depression, while most antidepressants are thought to potentiate transmission in biogenic amine synapses. It was therefore thought that depression arose from underactivity of certain central pathways for these amines, particularly noradrenaline and 5-HT.

There is evidence that the turnover of 5-HT in the brain is low in some patients with depression, as measured by levels of the metabolite 5-HIAA in the cerebrospinal fluid. This abnormality is linked to a risk of violent suicide attempts, and in other contexts to violent behaviour. For most patients, however, no differences in the metabolites are found; this has led to the view that the receptors for these transmitters may be abnormally insensitive in depression.

Depression is accompanied by abnormalities in neuroendocrine function, particularly raised levels of cortisol, resistance to suppression by dexamethasone, and blunting of the response of thyroid stimulating hormone to thyrotrophin releasing hormone. Pharmacological probes such as clonidine (alpha 2-agonist) and d-fenfluramine (releasing 5-HT) have been used to assess central NA and 5-HT receptor function, by measuring the release of growth hormone, prolactin, or cortisol evoked by the drug. The results suggest that there are indeed abnormalities in receptor function in depression, but these are elusive.

Critical features

Doctors judge the inappropriateness of depressed mood by comparing their patient's feelings and behaviour with those of others, and more especially with people who resemble that patient in sex, and ethnic and social backgrounds. If they know one of their patients, or have the advice of someone who does, they may decide the feeling and behaviour are inappropriate for that patient, because the patient is different from his/her individual norm, even though the difference does not fall outside the normal range for people of their sort. Some patients can recognise this finer degree of inappropriateness in themselves.

The more intense the depression the more likely it is to be associated with other symptoms, here termed the biological response – sleep disturbance, loss of appetite and weight, loss of all pleasurable response (anhedonia), loss of libido, loss of drive, fatigue, loss of interests, and impaired concentration. Psychomotor retardation or agitation may be recognised. Guilt and hopelessness, increased anxieties and obsessions colour the thought content. Hypochondriacal worries develop, and various depressive delusions and even hallucinations occur in psychotic depression. The mood itself may show a lack of reactivity to anything cheerful and may exhibit a diurnal variation, with the mood being worse in the morning. There may also be the wish to sleep for ever, for life to come to an end, and even the idea of ending life, and these thoughts must be asked for. The presence and severity of these symptoms, not necessarily all of them, in association with depressive feeling is a measure of the patient's psychobiological response, whether to external emotional stresses, or to internal bodily disturbances.

The more pronounced the biological response, the more likely physical methods of treatment will be necessary and helpful.

Some patients do not admit to depressed feelings. They may, however, be preoccupied with their physical and mental health. Their complaints may be of pains, headache, loss of all interest, inexplicable anxiety, fear of serious illness, or compulsive thoughts. Only when directly asked do they admit to psychobiological symptoms. These patients are examples of masked depression, to be treated with antidepressants or electroconvulsive therapy (ECT) like those with other depressive illnesses. Such patients may be first referred by their general practitioners to physicians and surgeons who must be aware that depression can masquerade as other illnesses.

Some patients are preoccupied by past failures. Depression sometimes seems reactive to life situations, especially loss events – loss of loved ones, loss of self-esteem through failures in work, the declining powers of middle-age, sudden misfortunes, sexual disappointments, and so on. Early loss of a parent may be relevant, and the adult may have difficulties when their own children reach the same age of the loss. At times, depression seems inexplicable.

But life stresses, whether present or absent, are irrelevant in deciding to use ECT or psychotropic drugs. It is not the supposed stress but the patient's biological responses to it which matter in choosing the treatment. Ignore presumed psychosocial causes and concentrate on the pattern of symptoms in deciding on drug management of the case. Always bear in mind the risk of suicide (see Appendix 3).

Recognition of the circumstances which provoke depressive illness indicate the focus for psychological and social help when the acute phase of the illness is over. These approaches are used more to strengthen the patient against future illness than to relieve the present one. General psychological support of the patient in hospital is important in lessening the patient's distress, but does not cure a severe illness. If there is no sustained improvement after ten days, it may be dangerous not to proceed with physical methods of treatment.

Depression associated with other conditions

People of less ability than their social manner indicates may find themselves in jobs or situations beyond their capacity and may become depressed by failure. People of abnormal personality get into scrapes which others avoid, and may become depressed by the consequences. People whose memories and intellectual capacities fail early, for instance in organic dementia before 60, may present with depression as their abilities diminish.

Depression can be an important symptom in conditions associated with brain damage, stroke, head injury, epilepsy, Parkinsonism, multiple sclerosis, rheumatoid arthritis and other chronic disabilities. Cancer, some endocrine disorders, vitamin deficiencies, and viral infections also seem to be associated with depression. Some drugs predispose to depression; others, if stopped after long use, may result in depression. Alcohol or substance abuse will contribute to depression and interfere with treatment.

The term 'secondary depression' is reserved for those cases in which depressive illness develops in the presence of another psychiatric or physical disorder. Such depression may therefore have psychological or physiological causes, and sometimes both. In such cases both the primary condition and the depression itself may need to be treated.

Classification of depression

Many attempts have been made to subdivide depressive illness into groups with distinctive treatments. These have proved of limited use in everyday practice. The older distinction between endogenous and reactive depression is replaced by the recognition that most depressions arise from an interaction of biological predisposition and psychosocial stress.

Depressive illnesses vary in severity, some showing a wider range or more intense symptoms than others; in general the mildest show less response to physical methods of treatment, and the most severe may have a poor long-term prognosis. The pattern of sleep disturbance guides whether a sedative drug should be used.

The recognition of agitation is important. If severe it is likely to require a sedative antidepressant or additional treatment with an antipsychotic such as chlorpromazine. A psychotic depression with delusions or hallucinations will often benefit more from a combination of an antidepressant with an antipsychotic than from either alone, and is also more likely to be drug-resistant and to need ECT.

The distinction between bipolar and unipolar patients is of some value as those with a bipolar history or family history are more likely to respond to lithium as an antidepressant.

The pattern of symptoms may be 'atypical'. This term is used to describe either those patients with a 'reversed functional shift', or those with prominent anxiety or panic. The reversed functional shift is common in patients with seasonal affective disorder who suffer winter depression. It involves hypersomnia, lethargy and increased appetite, especially for calorie-rich (carbohydrate) foods.

Early action

The first step, after having established a likely diagnosis of depression and explored the psychosocial context, is to offer the patient an explanation of their symptoms, sympathy and encouragement. Sometimes a single interview will help them to understand their problems better and leads to a resolution of the symptoms. This is more likely with an acute situational depression, or a depression without symptoms of biological response. It is less likely to apply to a patient referred after prior assessment by another doctor.

In the case of an acute situational depression, it is sometimes helpful to ensure a good night's sleep, using 10–30 mg temazepam or 25–l00 mg chlorpromazine in one dose. Size of dose depends on weight, age, physical health, and previous experience of the drug. It is better to achieve excessive sleep the first night and then reduce the dose, than to start with doses of small effect and then cautiously advance night by night. Control should be swift.

If there is anxiety or restlessness, day sedatives from once daily to four-hourly in severe cases will help in the short term. Here the dosage must be more cautious because of the risk of drowsiness, confusion and falling: single doses of diazepam (2–10 mg), oxazepam (10–30 mg), chlorpromazine (50 mg), or thioridazine (50 mg) may assist. Low doses of a sedative antidepressant can also be used. Relief of distress by day, like improvement of sleep by night, may start a general lifting of the depression and the drug may not be needed long in less severe cases. Many patients will prefer to avoid sedative medication if it carries a risk of dependence, as with benzodiazepines.

The depressed person often feels alone. Mustering the

concern of relatives and friends may be helpful. A temporary change of environment, such as staying with a friend, may bring some relief. Admission to hospital may relieve environmental anxieties and obligations but should not be rushed into. Admission may well be correct where there is a serious risk of suicide or of danger to others, or in cases of anti-social behaviour or a particularly unhelpful environment. On occasion, compulsory admission will be life-saving. However, the depressed person who is still working may not need to stop work, or have everyday social links and responsibilities taken away. Separation of mother and baby is usually bad for both (most hospitals now have mother and baby units).

The person with an acute depressive reaction, seemingly precipitated by some life event, and the mildly depressed person, particularly if obsessional, or where anxious or hypochondriacal symptoms are prominent, may improve in a few days and stay well simply with refreshing sleep and some daytime sedation. Likewise a patient admitted to hospital should be observed for up to one week with as little medication as possible, in order to clarify their symptom pattern and any response to non-specific treatment. During this time insomnia or daytime restlessness should be treated as above. If there is no improvement or the improvement is temporary, lasting say only 7–14 days, then specific treatment is indicated.

Specific treatment

The greater sureness and speed of electroconvulsive therapy (ECT) is valuable where for example the depression is severe or there is a risk of suicide, or it is urgent for a man to get back to work or a mother to return to young children. A psychotic depression will usually require ECT. However, the majority of patients should be treated firstly with antidepressants of the MARI class or – less commonly – an MAOI. The drawbacks of these drugs are their slow onset of action – taking up to ten days for improvement to begin, and four to six weeks for full effect – their side-effects, and, in some cases, their toxicity in overdose. These aspects should all be explained to the patient. They are then more likely to adhere to a treatment which they start. Drugs which are cardiotoxic in overdose should be avoided in patients with heart disease or who are a suicide risk; with the latter, steps should be taken to limit their access by prescribing for only one week at a time, or entrusting a relative to supervise the medication. While antidepressant medication is being taken it must be accompanied in virtually all cases by 'clinical management'. This includes educating the patient about the illness and its treatment, providing support, advice and encouragement, enlisting the help of others, relatives and community psychiatric nurses, guiding the patient regarding prognosis and assessing clinical state and suicide risk until recovery. In the longer term, selected patients may benefit additionally from exploring past and present relationships and roles in interpersonal psychotherapy, with the aim of improving their psychological adjustment. However, this approach alone is much less effective than medication and clinical management for the relief of depression. In general, psychobiological symptoms require physical treatment.

Antidepressants first became available in 1957 with the tricyclic antidepressant (TCA) imipramine investigated by Kuhn, and the MAOI iproniazid. In both cases their antidepressant effects were discovered by chance, in the course of their investigation as a tranquilliser or for tuberculosis. Newer antidepressants, such as fluoxetine, do not have a tricyclic structure but are grouped together with the older drugs under the name monoamine reuptake inhibitors (MARIs).

Of the tricyclic antidepressants, amitriptyline is sedative, imipramine less so, and desipramine and nortriptyline even less. These drugs have the advantage of having been widely used and having proven efficacy in a variety of settings. Their side-effects and interactions with other drugs are mostly known, and routine assays exist for measurement of their blood levels. Their antidepressant action is slow to begin, up to 10 days or more. Give 25 mg three times daily for two days, then 50 mg three times daily for 12 days. If there is no sign of improvement at this stage, and side-effects are insignificant, the dose can be increased to 75 mg and occasionally even to 100 mg three times daily. Be guided by the severity of side-effects in limiting dosage. In milder cases 100 mg daily may suffice. To control restlessness or anxiety a benzodiazepine or a phenothiazine can be added, in the doses quoted above, and used to control distress for a limited period only.

Patients metabolise and destroy drugs at varying rates, which is why different people require different doses. Laboratory measurement of plasma levels of antidepressant is occasionally helpful in adjusting dosage to avoid severe side-effects or poor therapeutic response.

Side-effects are worse in the first days of treatment, or just after each dose increase. The patient who has had the purpose and side-effects of the drug explained is more likely to tolerate a dry mouth and other side-effects without asking for the treatment to be changed. If postural hypotension is a problem, changing to nortriptyline may produce less.

The whole of a day's dose can be taken on one occasion if side-effects do not prevent it: the customary ritual three times daily has no other advantage because tricyclics have long half-lives. In fact, taking a large dose at night when the patient is lying down minimises the hypotensive and other side-effects; the patient is asleep when he might be experiencing them most. A single daily dose also aids adherence.

Newer monoamine reuptake inhibitors

These were developed in the hope of achieving faster onset of action, greater efficacy, fewer side-effects, and less cardiotoxicity. None have greater efficacy for depression in general; claims of faster action suggest that a drug has stimulant properties and that tolerance and dependence will develop. The new drugs are, however, much safer in overdose and have fewer autonomic side-effects. They include lofepramine, mianserin, trazodone, and the serotonin-specific reuptake inhibitors (SSRIs).

Monoamine oxidase inhibitors

These drugs are quite different from tricyclics in their mode of action and their value is less well-defined. Those hitherto available also carry special dangers and distinct dietary disadvantages. They may be effective for 'atypical depressions', in which depressive feelings co-exist with severe anxiety or panic, hypochondriacal complaints or a reversed functional shift with lethargy, fatigue, increased sleep and increased food intake. Insomnia, if present, is not of the early-waking type and depressive delusions are absent.

MAOIs are slower to act on mood than MARIs but occasionally produce impressive results in typical as well as atypical cases, especially those with pronounced anxiety. Phenelzine has been the most commonly prescribed. Tranylcypromine and isocarboxazid are useful alternatives. The effect of these irreversible MAOI drugs continues for up to four weeks after the patient has stopped taking them, the time required to synthesise fresh enzyme to replace that inactivated by the drug. This is important because the interaction with tyramine produces the 'cheese reaction' and the interaction with clomipramine and the SSRIs produces the 'serotonin syndrome' which is potentially fatal (see p. 56).

Moclobemide is the first of a new class of drugs, the reversible inhibitors of monoamine oxidase A (RIMA). It has a much smaller interaction with foodstuffs and with other drugs, and being reversible the risk of an interaction with SSRIs lasts only for a few days after it is stopped.

MARI-resistant depression

If amitriptyline, imipramine or dothiepin in the maximum tolerated doses of up to 300 mg per day for a month do not work, changing to another tricyclic is not likely to improve matters. Adding lithium carbonate to the tricyclic may produce an improvement sometimes within a few days. Likewise lithium carbonate may be added to an SSRI with benefit. Otherwise a complete change of medication is indicated, or ECT used. ECT is compatible with MARI treatment and, where MARIs alone have failed, ECT may succeed. Their combined use can produce the best result for severe depression.

ECT is the most effective treatment for resistant depression because of its speed of response and rate of success as compared with drugs. It is safe, suitable for the pregnant, the over-80s, those with healed coronary infarcts and other physical illnesses. Advice on technique, how many treatments to give, and how to judge improvement, is given at the end of the book. With ECT given alone, patients may relapse within two weeks; this may be avoided by continuing with a MARI in the long term.

For psychotic depression the combination of an MARI with an antipsychotic such as chlorpromazine is often necessary. There is a pharmacokinetic interaction, increasing the level of the tricyclic (see p. 16). The antipsychotic flupenthixol is thought to have some antidepressant properties when used alone and may be of use in less severe cases.

Occasionally lithium alone is useful as an antidepressant. The patients most likely to benefit are those with a history or family history of mania and those 'atypical' depressions with a reversed functional shift. These include patients with seasonal affective disorder and winter depression. In the latter, MAOIs and MARIs are sometimes effective. Phototherapy with extra exposure to bright light for an hour each day, at the beginning or end of the day to extend the daylight period, also helps to alleviate the condition.

When MAOIs and MARIs separately have failed, an MAOI and a tricyclic in combination may work. The combination is potentially dangerous because of the risk of the 'serotonin syndrome', or hypotension. Clomipramine or the SSRIs must not be combined with an MAOI. However, certain combinations are safer, for instance, amitriptyline or imipramine with phenelzine, tranylcypromine or moclobemide. The tricyclic antidepressant is usually started first, but the drugs may be started together – the MAOI in the morning and the tricyclic in the evening to make best use of any sedative effect (see p. 212). Phenelzine and amitriptyline are commonly used. Low blood pressure and other combination side-effects must be looked for. The treatment is therefore best started in hospital where good observation is possible. Otherwise, the patient should be seen every second or third day as an out-patient.

The doses of tricyclic drug and MAOI may be increased, depending on symptom response and side-effects, in small increments to the maximum dose levels of each, as if used on its own. Tranylcypromine in such combinations is particularly associated with side-effects of hypotensive faints, headache and insomnia.

L-tryptophan, 3–6 g daily, was useful as an adjunct to MAOI or tricyclic, and lithium was added in triple therapy. Tryptophan has now been withdrawn because of the occurrence of the eosinophilia-myalgia syndrome which is thought to be caused by a contaminant in the production of L-tryptophan. It is still available for use on a 'named patient' basis. The addition of a small dose of triiodothyronine (T_3) (25 µg) to a tricyclic has been shown to augment the antidepressant effect; this may be tried in selected cases, and continued as long as the tricyclic.

Outcome

Antidepressant drugs begin by suppressing symptoms rather than abolishing the underlying malfunction. If the drugs are stopped as soon as the patient has lost all symptoms, relapse is likely. After four weeks of being well the dose may be reduced, the return of symptoms being looked for. Then continue the drug for about six months more, albeit with reducing dosage, to allow time for the illness to resolve, whether by natural remission or from drug action. Do not reduce the dose just as the patient leaves hospital, or resumes his job, or is exposed to special stress. Choose a socially stable and quiet time. Too early cessation of drugs may result in an avoidable relapse, discouraging to the patient, the family and the employer.

Treatment failure

Among patients with depressive illness about one-third will improve without specific treatment and one-third will remain depressed after a course of antidepressants. The alternative treatments described above reduce this proportion. Nevertheless, physical treatments are not always effective. For the depressed patient who remains ill, try to identify the area of failure. Was the right dose prescribed? Did the patient take the drug as instructed? Did the side-effects prevent a high enough dose being achieved? If so, try a different drug of the same family or a slower build-up to a bigger dose. Were therapeutic levels ever achieved? Lack of side-effects may be a pointer to failure here. The effects of phenytoin, carbamazepine and other drugs concurrently taken may decrease drug levels. Laboratory measurements help to decide if plasma levels are within the therapeutic range. If levels are too low, try just exceeding the recommended upper dose limit; if too high a lower dose may work. Were benzodiazepines or anticonvulsant drugs being taken while ECT was given, and suppressing a fit?

Has the symptom pattern changed, even though recovery is incomplete? For example, the treatment may have caused a switch from depression to hypomania; abolished the biological symptoms of a depressive illness but with the patient retaining the sick role and exhibiting anxiety symptoms; or depressive symptoms may have cleared, leaving an unsuspected dementia with consequent inadequacies of function.

Failure of treatment should lead to review of the diagnosis. Is there an unrecognised medical illness? Thyroid disease in particular should be excluded. Is there a neurosis or personality disorder as well as depression? Is there a problem with alcohol or substance abuse? Are there marital difficulties undermining recovery?

A planned programme of drugs and ECT, with the treatment and response recorded, enables a confident conclusion about the effectiveness or otherwise of each, in defined dose and circumstance. The record is invaluable because the failed treatments need not then be tried again in later episodes, avoiding unneeded suffering. Sometimes a second course of ECT is more effective than the first, perhaps because the illness has reached a different stage.

Most depressive illnesses recover spontaneously, even after years. When depression is not too distressing or handicapping, waiting is probably the best course. But can the patient wait? Is the distress too severe or the risk of suicide too great? Be prepared to refer to a colleague interested in affective disorders. Leucotomy, now rarely used, may provide relief in these less common circumstances.

Even the most effective drug treatment does not usually restore to full health immediately. A return to complete personal and social competence may take many months after removal of the most distressing and disabling symptoms. Sometimes, reversion to pre-illness health is never achieved, leaving a deficit which can last indefinitely. Attempts to treat the deficit may cause more harm than good.

Preventing further illness

One depressive illness indicates a risk of further attack or attacks. There may be years of health before the illness recurs, or only a few months. A third episode may follow the second after a shorter time, and a fourth come sooner still. What can be done to prevent attacks or reduce their severity?

Prophylaxis by physical treatment is only appropriate where the illness recurs frequently (say within three years or less).

The agents of proven value in recurrent unipolar depression are the MARIs and lithium. Amitriptyline, dothiepin, nortriptyline, imipramine, sertraline and probably other MARIs prevent the recurrence of depression. They should be used in the same dose found effective for the patient's episode of acute depression. Because they appear to predispose to mania, MARIs should not be used alone for prophylaxis of bipolar disorder, but with lithium (see p. 229). Patients with recurrent depression most likely to benefit from lithium are those with stable personality, good inter-episode functioning and a family history of mania or of response to lithium. A steadily maintained plasma level of 0.5–1.0 mmol/l of lithium is needed. When an illness is periodically recurrent, perhaps seasonal, to start or stop anti-manic and antidepressant drugs in tune with its rhythm may only emphasise it. A long-term plan of prevention is better, and psychological methods have a place in prophylaxis besides drugs.

Further reading

ELKIN, I., SHEA, T. M., WATKINS, J. T., *et al* (1989) National Institute of Mental Health Treatment of Depression, Collaborative Research Programme. General effectiveness of treatments. *Archives of General Psychiatry*, **46**, 971–982.

JOFFE, R. T., SINGER, W., LEVITT, A. J., *et al* (1993) A placebo-controlled comparison of lithium and triiodothyronine augmentation of tricyclic antidepressants in unipolar refractory depression. *Archives of General Psychiatry*, **50**, 387–393.

KUHN, R. (1958) The treatment of depressive states with C.22355 (Imipramine hydrochloride). *American Journal of Psychiatry*, **115**, 459.

KUPFER, D. J., FRANK, E., PEREL, J. M., *et al* (1992) Five-year outcome for maintenance therapies in recurrent depression. *Archives of General Psychiatry,* **49**, 769–773.

QUITKIN, F. M., HARRISON, W., STEWARD, J. W., *et al* (1991) Response to phenelzine and imipramine in placebo non-responders with atypical depression. *Archives of General Psychiatry,* **48**, 319–323.

9 Mania

Overtalkativeness, overactivity, and overcheerfulness are the cardinal signs of mania, and increased irritability, flight of ideas, distractibility, and a failure of judgement may be obvious too. Grandiosity and decreased need for sleep complete the picture. Irritability leads to verbal and even physical aggression; exasperation with imposed restraints leads to feelings of persecution. Distractibility results in a changeable temper. Lack of judgement may cause irresponsible, impetuous acts which may be criminal or socially unacceptable. A previously well-conducted person may start to drink heavily, get involved in fights, or become promiscuous. In the milder forms, racing thoughts and cheerfulness, without outwardly visible pressure of talk or overactivity, may be the only abnormalities. Sometimes, those who know the patient can see they are unwell even though talk, mood and activity seem within the normal to strangers (hypomania).

Manic attacks may develop slowly taking some days, or rapidly over a few hours. They may start from a normal state or follow a depressive illness. They may succeed psychological stress, surgery or infection, or follow childbirth, or the use of antidepressants, electroconvulsive therapy (ECT) or other drugs, especially steroids or stimulants. They may result from discontinuation of drugs, especially lithium. Some are seasonal, occurring more often in the summer. This suggests diverse aetiologies leading to a common symptom expression. However, all are managed on the same principles. Attacks may last a few days or weeks but usually continue for months, ending sometimes without treatment. Most patients with mania suffer at other times with episodes of depression and are called BP (Bipolar)-I. Unipolar mania is less common and otherwise resembles bipolar mania. Some patients with recurrent depression have hypomanic episodes not requiring admission and are called BP-II.

Mania can affect people of all social and occupational groups. Hypomanic traits and episodes can be associated with successful leadership, productivity and creativity. Manic episodes are very disruptive and can be socially disastrous and there is a high rate of divorce and suicide in bipolar patients.

Treatment has three aims:

(a)   managing the patient and the problems created by manic conduct
(b)   controlling with drugs the abnormal mental state and behaviour including any depressive or mixed phase following mania
(c)   preventing further attacks.

Managing the patient

Do not argue with the patient – humour him, attempt to establish rapport by discussing the changes he will have noticed, his lack of sleep, his difficulties with family and friends and at work. Use these as the grounds on which he needs your help, possibly with drugs. Maintain gentle, calm friendly handling, steering him away from extravagant behaviour and indiscretion. Explain to the family that mania is an illness which causes a temporary restlessness, loss of judgement and sense of proportion, from which recovery is expected, so that they may be tolerant and forgiving, avoiding challenges.

In the first episode the family will need much counselling. Mania is the most genetic and often the most insightless form of mental illness. Most manic episodes are best treated in hospital, not only to give family and society relief from a trying responsibility, but also to avoid long-term damage to career and marriage. Much skill is needed in achieving this by persuasion. Compulsory admission under the Mental Health Act may be the best method with severe cases, because of refusal to accept treatment or because of the likelihood of poor adherence to drug treatment out of hospital or, indeed, in it.

In hospital, give as much living space as possible; confinement breeds conflict. Two manic patients on a ward can cause chaos. It may be necessary to prevent use of the telephone, to remove cheque books and credit cards, warn the bank, stop car driving and ban business engagements. The patient's demands can be seemingly endless. If you remain firm on limits understood and agreed by staff, family and associates, patients usually accept them. They may not understand the restrictions but, provided you remain friendly and calm, they may follow them to please you. The less cooperative patient needs either individual attention or nursing in a locked intensive care ward to prevent them from leaving.

Pathophysiology

The effects of drug treatment suggest that mania involves overactivity of certain central DA (and NA) pathways and underactivity of certain ACh and 5-HT pathways. There is limited direct biochemical evidence to support this view. The role of other transmitters and neuromodulators is not known.

Drug treatment of mania

Mild mania may be treated with antipsychotic drugs such as haloperidol 5–15 mg daily. Lithium treatment is also useful but improvement takes one to two weeks. Moderate or severe mania is usually most rapidly controlled by antipsychotic drugs. Phenothiazines (e.g. chlorpromazine) and thioxanthenes (e.g. zuclopenthixol) are effective but the butyrophenone, haloperidol, is often particularly useful in a dose of 5–10 mg three times a day. The more disturbed patient may be given haloperidol (5–10 mg) intramuscularly at two-hourly intervals until they are calm. Haloperidol (5–10 mg) may also be given intravenously. Larger intramuscular doses (e.g. 30 mg) are discouraged because they are excessive in some patients, and because their effect may last for several days, obscuring the diagnosis and making further management difficult; the patient may no longer appear very disturbed but is likely to deteriorate unless treatment is continued.

Haloperidol tends to produce initial sedation which wears off after a day or so during continued treatment. If the patient remains very behaviourally disturbed, chlorpromazine or zuclopenthixol may be more useful because they are more sedative than haloperidol. However, many manic patients resent being made to feel drowsy and this limits the doses they will accept. Chlorpromazine is hypotensive and should be used cautiously in the elderly.

Extrapyramidal side-effects, particularly dystonia, seem less of a problem with larger doses of haloperidol, but may emerge as the dose is reduced or some days after it is discontinued. Anti-Parkinsonian medication should therefore be continued for at least seven days after haloperidol is stopped.

Rapid improvement in mania occurs for one to three days after starting medication, and more gradually over the next two weeks. There is no evidence that increasing the dose of haloperidol above 30 mg per day achieves greater long-term improvement. Generally the more sedative drugs do not produce greater long-term improvement than less sedative ones.

For manic patients whose failure to improve is due to poor compliance, depot antipsychotic medication including haloperidol can be used. The acetate of zuclopenthixol is a depot formulation ('Acuphase') which has a duration of action of up to three days and a more rapid onset than the decanoates. It is useful in very disturbed patients who persistently refuse oral medication, during the first few days of treatment (see p. 251).

Other sedative drugs

For those who are not adequately sedated by antipsychotic drugs, or to avoid such drugs, sedation may be achieved by a benzodiazepine such as diazepam (10–20 mg intravenously or 30 mg orally). For intramuscular use, midazolam is absorbed faster and causes less local pain. Lorazepam (6–24 mg daily) can also be used alone or as an adjunct to other anti-manic drugs for short-term treatment. Depersonalisation and dissociation are potential problems with benzodiazepines, and, in the longer term, dependence and withdrawal symptoms.

Neuroleptic-resistant mania

A proportion of patients show only partial improvement or initial improvement followed by partial relapse with antipsychotic drugs. The main alternatives or adjuncts to the antipsychotics are lithium and the anticonvulsants, carbamazepine and valproate.

Lithium

About 60% of manics show a good response to lithium which usually requires two weeks to approach the full effect on mania. Used alone it is more useful in mild than in severe cases. Patients who respond tend to be classical manics rather than mixed or schizoaffective states. Patients who have benefited previously from lithium are more likely to do so again. Those in a rapid-cycling phase tend not to respond to lithium.

Doses in acute mania

The narrow gap or overlap between therapeutic and toxic blood levels of lithium necessitates careful monitoring of blood levels, usually based on samples taken 12 hours after the last dose. Increasing plasma levels of lithium above 0.8 mmol/l up to 1.4 mmol/l are associated with higher rates of response in mania, but levels above 1.2 mmol/l require special care in monitoring to avoid toxicity. When a suitable patient does not respond at a lower dose it is necessary to increase the level to the top of the therapeutic range before concluding that the individual is non-responsive. Many of the features of toxicity may reflect high intracellular rather than extracellular levels; hence, in assessing toxicity and efficacy, clinical judgement rather than blood levels should be paramount.

Lithium-neuroleptic combinations

Combinations of high levels of lithium with high doses of antipsychotics including haloperidol have been associated with severe neurological symptoms resembling lithium toxicity, perhaps because antipsychotic drugs can increase intracellular lithium levels. It is generally safe to combine haloperidol (up to 30 mg daily) with lithium at levels of up to 1 mmol/l. Thus, when combining these treatments, the blood levels should generally be maintained below 1 mmol/l; staff should be advised to observe and report the development of neurological symptoms, and lithium should be temporarily discontinued if they develop.

Carbamazepine

Carbamazepine is approximately as effective as lithium, with about 60% of patients doing well. There is some delay in its action but less so than with lithium. More severely ill manic patients including mixed or dysphoric manics can benefit from carbamazepine, and a history of non-response to lithium does not reduce the chances of responding to carbamazepine. Patients with no family history of mania may have a greater chance of responding, and mania secondary to brain damage can also benefit.

The dose of carbamazepine used in acute mania is similar to that used for epilepsy except that the starting dose has to be less gradual to avoid delay. Starting with 400 mg daily, the dose can be increased according to response and side-effects to a maximum of 1600 mg daily. Blood tests should be monitored (see p. 290).

Valproate in acute mania

Valproate is effective in a proportion of manic patients including non-responders to antipsychotic drugs, lithium and carbamazepine. Most of the improvement occurs within days of achieving therapeutic levels (15–100 mg/l). The drug is generally well tolerated but side-effects include tremor, weight gain, rash, transient hair loss and, potentially, acute liver damage. Liver function tests should be monitored. The starting dose is 600 mg daily, rising to 2000 mg according to clinical response.

Combination treatment

Many patients who fail to improve when taking carbamazepine alone do so when lithium is added. This combination – as with neuroleptics – increases the risk of lithium neurotoxicity. Carbamazepine can also be combined with valproate but pharmacokinetic interactions occur and more careful monitoring of dose is needed.

Use of ECT in mania

Many clinicians reserve ECT for only the most severe and drug-resistant manic patients, and it is possible that more widespread use would be justified. In early reports, about two-thirds of patients given ECT in mania showed marked improvement. In a double-blind trial, ECT was superior to lithium during the first eight weeks, especially for severe mania and for mixed states.

Follow-up

The return of a patient's mental state to apparent normality does not allow lessening of clinical vigilance. Within hours or days a swing into a dangerous (suicidal) depressive state may occur. Equally, severe extrapyramidal side-effects may suddenly develop. Also the picture may change subtly with irritability and a mixed affective state, heralding the development of depression. These call for a reduction or even cessation of antipsychotic drugs, while continuing a mood-stabiliser, and considering an antidepressant.

Prophylaxis of bipolar disorder

Selection of patients

Maintenance treatment should be considered after a second episode of bipolar disorder, especially if the interval between episodes was less than five years. Because the intervals between the first and second episodes tend to be longer than between subsequent episodes, maintenance treatment should only be used after a first episode if the dangers of a subsequent episode are thought to justify it – for instance if the episode was severe and disruptive, had a relatively sudden onset and was not precipitated by external factors, or if the person's job is very sensitive, or there is a risk of suicide.

Lithium maintenance

Patients with typical bipolar disorder having complete recovery between episodes, or a family history of bipolar disorder, are more likely to benefit. Patients with a rapid-cycling phase of illness are less responsive to lithium. Other factors mitigating against prophylactic efficacy are poor adherence to treatment and drug abuse. A large proportion of patients at risk do not seek treatment, and many who do adhere poorly to lithium. There is also the risk of withdrawal mania in those who stop treatment too abruptly, for instance when feeling no need for it during a mild upswing of mood. However, where steps are taken to encourage and check adherence, low relapse rates and affective morbidity on lithium can be achieved. This is part of the rationale for specialist lithium or affective disorder clinics.

Patients are less likely to adhere if they are younger, male and have had fewer previous episodes. The reasons they give for stopping are drug side-effects, missing periods of elation, feeling well and in no need of treatment, feeling depressed or less productive, or not wanting to depend on medication. The side-effects most often given as reasons are excessive thirst and polyuria, tremor, memory impairment and weight gain.

In order to increase adherence, the doctor should take side-effects seriously, keep lithium levels as low as possible, educate the patients and their families about their illness and the use of lithium, and discuss adherence with the patient. Regular contact and counselling can be useful. It may be helpful to plot a 'life chart' with the patient.

Lithium lessens both the severity and the frequency of episodes. Usually it also stabilises the mood between major episodes. But only 60–70% of patients benefit. The mortality rate (high because of suicides) can be reduced on lithium to that of the general population.

Blood levels and monitoring

Blood levels lower than those formerly used are sufficient in prophylaxis (0.5–1.0 mmol/l). For some patients lower levels than this would suffice. In the elderly a level of 0.5 mmol/l is recommended. During less stable phases lithium levels should be done frequently, and even in the most stable, the tests of lithium level, renal and thyroid function should be done at least once a year.

Antidepressants and lithium

Depression occurring during lithium treatment can be treated with MARIs. In patients with BP-I disorder the course of antidepressant treatment should be gradually discontinued as the depression improves, in order to reduce the risk of triggering a manic episode and to avoid the induction of rapid cycling.

For patients with a predominantly depressive pattern of bipolar disorder (BP-II) the combination of lithium and a MARI may be more effective in preventing depression than either drug alone.

Withdrawal of lithium

Symptoms of anxiety, irritability and emotional lability can occur following sudden discontinuation. Abrupt cessation of lithium in bipolar patients leads to the development of mania two to three weeks later in up to 50% of patients. Discontinuation should therefore be gradual.

Patients whose mood has been stable are less likely to relapse on stopping than those who have continued to show mild mood swings. Lithium may be reduced at the rate of one-quarter to one-eighth of the original dose every two months.

Alternatives to lithium in maintenance

Even in favourable clinical trials, lithium maintenance was unsuccessful in over 30% of patients. About two-thirds of patients show good responses to carbamazepine. In contrast to lithium, rapid-cycling patients benefit as much from carbamazepine as do other patients. In longer-term use there may be partial loss of efficacy by the third year although it is not clear to what extent poor adherence to medication is responsible.

Side-effects of carbamazepine can be minimised by commencing treatment with low doses (100–200 mg at night) and increasing every few days to the maximum dose that is well tolerated (usually 400–600 mg, maximum 1600 mg daily). Patients should be informed of the risk of side-effects including blood disorders (see p. 290), and told to report to the doctor possible symptoms such as sore throat, rash or fever.

Some patients benefit more from the combination of lithium and carbamazepine than from either drug alone. There have been reports of reversible neurological side-effects characterised mainly by confusional states and cerebellar signs similar to those of lithium toxicity.

Sodium valproate has been studied less but can be useful in those who are resistant to lithium or carbamazepine. The combination of lithium with valproate produces fewer neurological problems than the combination of lithium and carbamazepine.

Antipsychotic drugs should be avoided if possible for long-term use in bipolar patients because of sedative effects and tardive dyskinesia. However, for those who have frequently recurring episodes and either do not benefit from or do not adhere to oral medication, depot antipsychotic medication can provide a period of stability.

Resistant bipolar disorders attract polypharmacy leading to the creation of a drug fog. Fear of relapse prevents attempts to reduce overmedication. A sensible course is admission, to remove at least some medicines by stages, and to review the value of others. If possible in such cases try to limit medication to mood-stabilising drugs and an antipsychotic or an antidepressant.

For a few patients a community psychiatric nurse, or day hospital attendance may prevent long admissions to hospital, but, for a minority, long-term hospital or hostel care is required.

Manic–Depressive Fellowship

This organisation offers advice and a regular newsletter, and has self-help groups in some areas.
13 Rosslyn Road, Twickenham, Middlesex, TW1 2AR.
Telephone: 081 892 2811.

Further reading

GOODWIN, F. K. & JAMISON, K. R. (1990) *Manic–Depressive Illness.* Oxford: Oxford University Press.

10   Schizophrenia

Patients with schizophrenia may show a great variety of behavioural and subjective symptoms and signs. A given individual may only suffer a selection of them, and symptoms may be different at different times in the course of the illness. Thus there may be inactivity and withdrawal from others and the environment in general, restlessness and emotional fluctuations to extremes of panic or suspicion, inappropriate laughter or sadness, the experience of auditory and tactile hallucinations, the expression of delusional ideas, and thinking may be clearly derailed.

Positive and negative symptoms

It is helpful to separate the symptoms of schizophrenia into positive symptoms (which cause abnormality by their presence), negative symptoms (which represent the absence of normal function), and symptoms of general psychopathology (which include depression and anxiety).

Positive symptoms are mainly delusions, hallucinations, illogical thinking and affective incongruity. The negative symptoms include poverty of speech, flatness of affect and a lack of drive. These are the 'core' negative symptoms, but other 'secondary' negative symptoms such as lack of self-care, social withdrawal, and muteness can develop in response to positive symptoms. Other negative symptoms can also develop as a result of understimulation, for instance in households or wards where there is a lack of personal interaction or activities, or in a barren environment. Overstimulation in an emotionally charged environment can also worsen the condition.

Antipsychotic drugs are very useful in alleviating positive symptoms and signs, but they are not curative, and form only part of the modern management of the illness. They are important in four circumstances:

(a)   emergency control of acute disturbance
(b)   relief of many of the symptoms in early phases or relapses
(c)   continuing reduction of symptoms in the chronically ill
(d)   prevention of recurrence of illness in those who have largely recovered.

In long-term care (c and d above) it becomes very evident that the negative symptoms are much less affected by drugs. Emotional flatness and indifference, inertia and anergy, and poverty of interest and responsiveness persist in the form of a defect state after recovery from an acute illness. They may then form the major disability in a chronically ill patient, and can be responsible for an otherwise normal-seeming person being unable to work or maintain social relationships.

A clinical interview lasting 60 minutes may not reveal either active symptoms or, even more, the negative defect state. Therefore independent accounts from those who see the patient every day, indicating how he/she has been behaving in different situations, may be essential to a good assessment. This points also to the need to advise and help the family to cope with the patient at home.

Sufferers can hide symptoms either deliberately, for example when paranoid, or from indifference and poor concentration in replying to questions. Conversely, certain stress situations, such as fatigue, criticism, presumed antagonisms, or strange experiences, evoke fears of inability to cope with the world and an acute exacerbation of positive symptoms results. Stresses on an individual may vary from day to day or hour to hour but, because of their illness, schizophrenic people have an abnormal sensitivity to such events which render them more vulnerable. Psychotropic drugs appear to lessen this sensitivity.

Neuropharmacology of schizophrenia

There is an important genetic contribution although this is less in those with a later age of onset. Chronic schizophrenia is associated with increased ventricular volume and reduced brain size. This is especially so in the temporal lobe where the hippocampus is small and shows abnormal cellular architecture, thought to be a developmental defect arising in foetal or neonatal life from genetic factors, virus infection or obstetric complications. The cortex is diminished in volume especially on the left side and near the speech areas.

According to the dopamine hypothesis, schizophrenia results from a functional overactivity of dopamine at certain synapses in the brain. The hypothesis is founded upon two observations.

Firstly, drugs which stimulate dopamine pathways, such as amphetamines or direct dopamine agonists such as bromocriptine, can produce psychosis resembling paranoid schizophrenia when taken in large doses.

Secondly, all known antipsychotic drugs have in common the ability to block dopamine receptors. However, there is little direct evidence in support of this hypothesis. Post-mortem studies show subtle changes in levels of dopamine and its metabolites in the brain. Dopamine receptor numbers are increased at post-mortem, but this may be entirely the result of previous exposure to antipsychotic drugs. Dopamine receptor numbers in the brains of unmedicated schizophrenic patients measured by positron emission tomography show no consistent increase, although there is some abnormal asymmetry with greater receptor numbers on the left side.

The disturbed patient

Aggressive or disturbed behaviour is now the usual reason for admitting patients with schizophrenia to hospital. Anaesthetisation with barbiturates, bromide, or morphine and hyoscine used to be all that was possible. With modern drugs, targets for suppression are hostility and dangerous behaviour, irritability and restlessness, but without reducing consciousness (see Chapter 11 – The violent patient). The drugs used in early treatment are given in larger doses, as syrup or by intramuscular, occasionally even by intravenous, injection. Chlorpromazine (50–100 mg), droperidol or haloperidol (10–20 mg), all given orally or intramuscularly, every two to four hours, should achieve rapid control within one to two days. Rarely, in a crisis, intravenous droperidol or haloperidol (10 mg) can be used. By the third or fourth day, as the patient improves, regular oral medication, syrup or tablets, should suffice. The changeover to oral doses requires care. A common error is to start off well and then lose control again through inadequate dosage. Start the oral drug while continuing but gradually lessening the injected doses and frequency. Careful monitoring of change is required for the ensuing two to three weeks. After absorbing large quantities of drug during an acute phase, patients may suddenly develop marked side-effects, such as drowsiness or acute dystonic reactions. The latter can be mistaken for symptoms of the illness. Anti-Parkinsonian drugs may be needed, at times by injection, and antipsychotic drugs reduced.

Treatment of early phases or relapses

This may be in hospital or at home. For those who refuse treatment, a compulsory admission may be appropriate if their condition meets the criteria for a section of the Mental Health Act (see Appendix 1). Patients often improve considerably once away from the stresses of home and ordinary life, particularly if the hospital offers a simple, calm routine. Through their illness they may suffer doubts and confusions about themselves, the world, and their relation to others; emotional relations with mother and father may be particularly upsetting. A clear structure for a basic daily pattern of activities, including getting up, washing, shaving, using make-up, and other self-care, meals and manageable tasks, either domestic or occupational therapy, helps them to return to reality and feel more effective. Permissiveness, on the contrary, may engender further confusion.

One or two nurses must make a special effort to befriend the patient; the establishment of a relationship even though, at times, seemingly tenuous, superficial or difficult, is always therapeutic provided it does not become too close. This means that the ward staff must have a constancy from day to day and week to week and not be subject to frequent posting, and they must be correctly identifiable by patients.

The building of confidence allows the patient to enter positively into the life of the ward and to cooperate with treatment, largely free of attacks of distress or violence. These objectives apply also to those treated in a day hospital or as out-patients, but efforts may be needed to persuade regular attendance. Supervision, by regular visiting from a community psychiatric nurse, is an invaluable part of out-patient treatment and allows for family and friends to report progress or setbacks.

Initial assessment of the patient means: (a) making sure that the illness falls in the schizophrenic group and is not an acute brain syndrome or an atypical manic–depressive disorder, for which the treatment and prognosis are different; (b) identifying symptoms – delusions, hallucinations, passivity feelings, poor concentration, paranoid thinking – which can be targets for medication, the subsequent decline of symptoms serving as a guide to further treatment and dosage; (c) judging whether the immediate prognosis is good from the acuteness of onset, the precipitating stresses including the taking of illicit drugs (amphetamines, cannabis, khat, etc.) and the presence of affective and other positive symptoms; (d) identifying family or social factors which may assist or retard recovery.

If the patient is not distressed or agitated, give a non-sedative antipsychotic such as trifluoperazine (10 mg, twice daily), haloperidol (5–10 mg, twice daily), sulpiride (400 mg, twice daily), or remoxipride (150–300 mg, daily). Within one or two weeks it should be clear whether the symptoms are lessening. If not, raise the dose gradually and review weekly. In the distressed or agitated patient, more sedative drugs are used. Start with chlorpromazine or thioridazine (100 mg, twice daily) or zuclopenthixol (10 mg, twice daily), again for one or two weeks, and then review. With experience, one learns to gauge from the severity of illness the dosage that will probably be required and to increase it by steps.

However, these drugs set in train a process of recovery which may not be obvious until two weeks have passed, and it takes four to eight weeks to achieve the full effect on positive symptoms. Further improvement may develop over the next year, especially if the patient has been ill for a long time before treatment and must regain neglected skills. During this time nothing is gained by increasing the dose of medication above a certain level (for instance above 20–30 mg a day for trifluoperazine and haloperidol). Start with lower doses and build up gradually because side-effects, for instance hypotension and dystonic reactions, are more severe if time for adaptation is not allowed. If dystonia, Parkinsonism or akathisia develop, they should be treated with anticholinergic drugs and explained to the patient. As the patient improves, sedative drugs have little advantage over the less sedative ones, and less sedative drugs may be preferable and more acceptable to the patient.

Once improvement is marked, the daily drug dose should be continued, but, if side-effects occur, cautiously reduce by steps every two to three weeks, watching for the return of symptoms as a sign to reduce the dose no further.

Some patients unwilling to take tablets are prepared to drink syrup, which is more quickly and regularly absorbed, and cannot secretly be got rid of by a paranoid patient. To start with, all the day's dose can be given at night as 'sleeping medicine', which some patients will accept while refusing daytime drugs. More rarely, those who refuse tablets or syrup will be prepared to have intramuscular injections. With tablets by mouth, one can never be sure that the patient is taking them and this may be a reason when phenothiazines seem to fail in treatment. Even if the patient has not expressed concern, it is important to inquire after side-effects, but without alarming the patient.

Failure to treat schizophrenia successfully with phenothiazines commonly arises because: (a) the patient is not getting the drug; (b) the doctor has been overcautious and not prescribed big enough doses; (c) the doctor has not waited long enough (at least two weeks) for improvement; (d) the doctor is making a global assessment only of behavioural improvement instead of watching for the decline of individual symptoms (hallucinations becoming infrequent and less forceful, concentration improving, logicality returning, restlessness declining). Even if there is no global improvement, the drugs may have produced a change in the symptom pattern, which shows they are doing something and can perhaps be used to better effect in larger doses or on a different schedule or by a different route. Some patients who do poorly with phenothiazines, which are extensively metabolised, will do better with another class of drugs such as butyrophenones. In general, however, there is no evidence that one antipsychotic drug produces greater long-term therapeutic effect than another in adequate doses. If the patient seems not to improve, it may be because there is an admixture of affective symptoms – depressive, manic or mixed – or because they have a neuroleptic-resistant schizophrenia.

Depressive symptoms occur in acute schizophrenia but are less obvious than the psychotic ones. Often the depression is only 'revealed' when antipsychotic drugs have improved the psychosis. Severe depression may also appear for the first time in the post-psychotic phase, as the patient recognises how ill they have been and confronts their problems more realistically. The addition of an antidepressant such as imipramine can improve both the depression and the overall clinical state. Likewise lithium will help to reduce elation and other symptoms of mania. Carbamazepine has a similar role and both drugs may also reduce impulsive or aggressive behaviour in schizophrenia. About 50% of patients show a good response to neuroleptics and a further 25% show moderate improvement.

For neuroleptic-resistant schizophrenia, the first drug with proven advantage over others is clozapine (see p. 259). Because of the risk of agranulocytosis, weekly blood tests in a formal monitoring system are required. Both positive and negative symptoms benefit, but cognitive impairment does not. There is definite benefit in social functioning in 30–60% of such patients.

Risperidone (4–8 mg daily) has also some advantage over haloperidol, including improvement in positive and negative symptoms, depression and anxiety (see p. 261).

Early successful treatment is shown by modification of symptoms. Later assessment is by observing the patients' abilities to mix with others, to concentrate and to make realistic decisions, and their capacity to undertake work and persist at it. Observations of nurses, occupational therapists and relatives are essential here. Do not increase doses further when these improvements appear. Rarely, electroconvulsive therapy (ECT) is of value in those patients who, despite adequate neuroleptics, have persistent disturbing symptoms associated with destructive behaviour. Do not go beyond the maximum of five treatments unless improvement is clearly occurring. ECT by itself usually has only a temporary suppressant effect on symptoms. Combined with phenothiazines, the effects last longer but tend to disappear by three months. For these reasons, ECT is not often used unless the psychosis is very severe or the patient is suicidal. However, it is effective for cases of acute catatonia and acute thought disorder, or when there is also severe depression. Defect state disabilities are *not* helped by ECT.

After a first florid episode, drugs should be continued for one year. If the patient has remained well, the drugs should then be withdrawn and the patient observed carefully for 3–12 months for the return of symptoms. About 20% will not have a further episode.

If, however, the acute episode was a recurrence, then long-term treatment should be considered and depot medication encouraged.

Remember that a schizophrenic illness can have a disastrous effect on the course of a person's life, for instance the prospects of a career and marriage. Choose the time for managing without drugs with great care so that if, by ill chance, a relapse does occur, it will not fall at a critically upsetting time for the patient. For example, a student who has a schizophrenic breakdown in his final year should be carried through his exams and well into his first job before considering drug withdrawal.

Before discharge from hospital, a plan of aftercare should be made following an 'assessment of needs' in which the views of the general practitioner, CPN, social worker, relatives and other professionals contribute. This is formalised in the care programme for informal patients and in Section 117 of the Mental Health Act 1983 for patients who have been detained on a Treatment Order.

With lessening in-patient facilities, more patients are managed outside hospital, perhaps attending as day patients or being closely monitored as out-patients by CPNs. Counselling of the family to manage home relationships is then essential. But the principles of drug treatment remain the same. Then it is particularly important for the patient to be reviewed regularly, for example on a weekly basis at first, monthly later, and for someone who lives with the patient to be regularly asked about him or her.

Longer-term management

After a first episode of schizophrenia a minority of patients become completely well. Others continue to require drugs to suppress their hallucinatory experiences or their morbid suspicion of people around them, or may develop a post-psychotic depressive illness requiring antidepressant drugs. In others, the psychotic experiences remit but disabling residual symptoms persist and they remain at risk of relapses.

These residual symptoms are of three kinds. Most common is a lack of energy, a lack of drive and inability to think coherently: although expressing the best intentions and seemingly fit, the patient in the extreme case is quite unable to work, and in many less extreme cases cannot manage a day's work at normal speed. Second is the lack of feeling, particularly an indifference to or unawareness of the feelings of others: the graces of social behaviour are dropped. Third is a preoccupation with eccentric ideas which may force the patient and perhaps family, to live in a restricted or unusual way.

Most patients who continue on drugs because they would be worse without them will be living outside of hospital, 'in the community', leading some semblance of a normal life, some at work. Few will be symptom-free, most will have some dysfunction.

In assessing residual symptoms, the negative symptoms of the illness itself must be distinguished from similar symptoms that can be caused by drugs. Parkinsonian side-effects can cause slowness (hypokinesia) and mental dullness (bradyphrenia), which are reversible by anticholinergic drugs. Excessive doses of antipsychotics may produce drowsiness and inattention. The schizophrenic patient with clinical depression may express feelings in an affectively flat way, and the usual disturbances of sleep and appetite may be masked by antipsychotic medication. Nevertheless, they can benefit from antidepressants. Depression, anxiety or insomnia are often part of the prodrome of relapse and require an increase in antipsychotic medication. Over-stimulation in a highly charged emotional environment can worsen symptoms with either relapse or increased withdrawal. Understimulation tends to exacerbate negative symptoms.

Too many patients are found continuing on a multiplicity of drugs, for example an oral as well as a depot antipsychotic, benzodiazepine and anti-Parkinsonian drugs, perhaps an antidepressant as well, sometimes for years. Medication should not become a standard routine but be reviewed regularly and cut down on a rational basis. The antipsychotic drug itself, the mainstay of the drug regime, may have become inappropriate in dose or schedule. Very few patients require both oral and depot antipsychotics in long-term treatment and the tablets should be converted to depot equivalents and phased out. Anti-Parkinsonian drugs may no longer be necessary, having been started in other circumstances. Minor tranquillisers or antidepressants, useful at an earlier stage, may not be required. Trying out changes of the drug regime, while looking for behavioural change either good or bad in the patient, may be needed to demonstrate what the regime is actually doing.

Relapse prevention and depot medication

Long-term use of antipsychotics requires careful consideration. They can produce harmful or unpleasant effects, tardive dyskinesia for instance, weight gain and drowsiness. In some patients their therapeutic value may be doubtful. On the other hand, a schizophrenic illness can be so devastating that it is justifiable to go to great lengths to prevent or minimise it. A single attack of acute schizophrenia will not usually justify long-term drug treatment, whereas two attacks two years apart or less, or three attacks in five years almost certainly will.

Without medication, 60–70% of patients with chronic schizophrenia will relapse within one year of stopping medication, and 85% within two years. The most common time to relapse is the second three months after stopping. These figures are greatly reduced by drug treatment but 10% will still relapse each year even among those who adhere fully to treatment. Education of the patient and their family about the illness and its treatment will help to improve adherence and facilitate a therapeutic alliance.

For many patients the regular contact with a CPN provides the best hope, by encouraging adherence in a continuing relationship with a professional who can advise on local services, counsel about new problems, and detect the early stages of relapse.

Taking tablets several times a day without fail can be difficult. Tablets which need to be taken only once a day are easier, but better still are the long-acting depot injections of antipsychotics. To be given as depot injections, the drug must be highly potent and esterified with a long-chain fatty acid so that a month's dose can be dissolved in a volume of vegetable oil small enough to be given by deep intramuscular injection. The available drugs include fluphenazine, flupenthixol, clopenthixol, haloperidol and pipothiazine. A single injection every one to six weeks may suffice as maintenance treatment. Such long-term treatment not only suppresses symptoms but prevents future relapse.

Patients with schizophrenia are often completely unaware of their illness or indifferent to it. Consequently they may be diffident about taking the tablets regularly which are, in fact, beneficial, or they may not ask for a further prescription. They do not come to the doctor who must seek them out if care is to be maintained: patients tend not to turn up for appointments and, if this happens, doctor, nurse or social worker must go to them at home. Again this is where a personal relationship is important in achieving continuity of treatment. An attendance each month at a local clinic run by a CPN is most helpful.

The care of schizophrenics is a long-term job and the CPN, who is usually the key worker, will need the support of a regular medical review, not by a succession of junior doctors but by a responsible consultant accompanied by doctors in their training. These depot team reviews should be conducted at least once a year for even the most stable patients and at three- to six-monthly intervals for less stable patients. Often it is the consultant and general practitioner who are able to provide continuity of care over many years. This is because patients and their illnesses evolve and slowly change and the effects of drugs on them alter. Their families and friends should be regularly asked about their performance.

When reviewing long-term treatment, look back over the history, the early symptoms before treatment started, the early signs of relapse, the circumstances of the last admission, and evidence of previous relapses when the dose has been reduced below a certain level. After controlling a relapse it is possible to reduce medication gradually over the next two years. The most common dose of fluphenazine decanoate in a group of out-patients is 25 mg a fortnight. Younger male patients require more, whereas older patients or those who have been free of relapse for three years manage with less. A dose as low as 2 mg a week may then be beneficial. Remember that after reducing the dose of the depot, the blood level will not reach the new steady state until about three to six months later and relapses related to earlier dose reductions can occur up to 18 months afterwards.

Obviously the patient whose hallucinations and paranoid outbursts are controlled by drugs should continue to take them. A problem arises in the chronically disabled person, predominantly lacking in energy or feeling, whose residual symptoms are not helped appreciably by drugs. Should they be on long-term treatment? The answer lies in deciding whether their condition is static or whether their history shows episodes of worsening – patches of bizarre or disturbed behaviour or increased vagueness or bewilderment for instance – and whether there has been previous experience of the patient relapsing when medication was reduced further. In these patients, long-term treatment is helpful in preventing relapses, and allows many schizophrenics to function better.

In or out of hospital, the general management of schizophrenics should try to meet their disabilities. Regular encouragement and moderate stimulation keep them from regressing too far into inertia. They need human relationships but not very demanding ones, whether in work or domestic life. Emotional stress predisposes to further breakdowns and young schizophrenics may do better away from home. The families of schizophrenics often need a good deal of advice and support and a common complaint is that they are not told enough about their condition and treatment.

Specific behavioural techniques may be useful in patients with particular behavioural difficulties, for instance 'attention-focusing' for poverty of speech, relaxation training for screaming or aggressive behaviour, and 'overcorrection' for urinary incontinence or enuresis. Intensive psychosocial interventions can exacerbate schizophrenia especially in patients on low-dose medication. But training on medication management, symptom management, social problem-solving and skills of successful living can improve social adjustment provided the patient is on medication. Thus the skills of a multidisciplinary team are needed.

The best strategy for long-term drug treatment is to gradually reduce the dose of medication to the lowest which keeps the patient free of relapse. Attempts to discontinue medication and then watch for the earliest symptoms of relapse are generally less successful and place the patient at greater risk.

Current practice leads to many schizophrenic patients with continuing impairment living outside hospital. They are vulnerable to exploitation and social pressures, and may have difficulty making friends or finding social entertainment. They are often poor at looking after their own domestic and business interests, failing to shop and cook for themselves, or to claim money to which they are entitled. Collaboration with voluntary bodies, such as the National Schizophrenia Fellowship, can provide a network of support and advice to patients and their relatives. SANE (Schizophrenia: A National Emergency) offers telephone advice. A local clinic should keep a register of all schizophrenic patients in the area, whether resident or coming and going, and CPNs mark the dates they are seen and issue reminders for fresh contact. Patients should be given a card which shows the dates of each appointment and the dates medication is given. A balance has to be struck between interference in the life of the disabled and encouragement to further independence. On the other hand, there have been too many examples of schizophrenics losing contact with the psychiatric services, missing their medication and coming back into treatment only after being arrested.

Patients discharged from hospital often take time to recover their full capacity for self-government. Aftercare hostels should be available providing appropriate levels of support, and the hostel staff should work with the patient's key worker (usually the CPN) to plan the next stage of rehabilitation. Day centres and drop-in centres are useful in providing daytime activity at a level appropriate for the patient's needs.

National agencies

National Schizophrenia Fellowship, National Office: telephone 081 547 3937.
Advice line: telephone 081 974 6814.
SANE line: telephone 071 724 8000.

Further reading

BRADLEY, P.B. & HIRSCH, S.R. (1980) *The Psychopharmacology and Treatment of Schizophrenia.* Oxford: Oxford University Press.

11 The violent patient

Management

Violence is the exercise of physical force so as to cause injury or damage to oneself, others, or property. Aggression is the threat of violence.

A traditional way of coping with the violence of the mentally ill was by physical restraint: chains, the strait waistcoat, seclusion in the padded cell. Then, in the early 19th century, came the demonstration in England that calm, friendly concern for the individual and simple psychological management made much of restraint unnecessary. With the advent of drugs, morphine, hyoscine and the barbiturates became the compellers of peace, in effect by partial anaesthetisation. With modern, more subtle psychotropics which leave consciousness untouched, psychological handling has again become an important component of management. The violent patient presents the most extreme challenge to the psychiatrist of how to combine psychology and pharmacology in effective proportion, a balance which is also needed in the treatment of psychoses and neuroses in general.

In the general hospital ward the psychiatrist may be asked to help not only with the violent but in cases with lesser degree of disturbance, sometimes involving complex problems of diagnosis or management, and not necessarily to arrange removal of the patient. What the psychiatrist offers is:

(a)   a skill in gaining the patient's confidence and sensitivity to slight pointers in history or behaviour suggesting an organic as well as a psychological origin of symptoms

(b)   a systematic assessment of mental state, covering all main mental functions

(c)   pursuit of a detailed, reliable history, with awareness of the relevance of social and interpersonal factors on the one hand and of the toxic signs of medicines or illicit drugs on the other

(d)   the ability at times to wait and observe further before drawing conclusions

(e)   continuity of care, with only one doctor in charge and keeping medication to the minimum, and maintaining, with nurses, a clear and consistent approach to problems

(f)   involvement of relatives or friends in gaining the patient's confidence

(g)   keeping a record of medication and behavioural change.

Be wary of clever labels and glib interpretations. Be prepared to seek advice from colleagues with more experience. Spend time with nurses, who bear the brunt of difficult behaviour.

In the accident and emergency centre, violent and dangerous behaviour is common. Drunks and psychopaths are often quickly recognised and deflected towards the police. But beware of too ready use of such 'nuisance' labels and of overlooking mania, schizophrenia, drug-induced psychosis, head injury or post-epileptic state. With the latter, on careful examination, some degree of altered consciousness can be detected even if no history is available.

Procedure

Whatever the setting, it is important to have an adequate and defined space for the interview, so that the patient can move about and not feel restricted. Do not ignore the potentially violent person. It is essential that the doctor appears calm and neutral in manner and can adopt a relaxed, friendly stance. Speak calmly and in a low tone.

Non-verbal communication matters. Try to establish a relationship of trust; allow them to verbalise their concerns. Do not promise anything that cannot be carried out, and if it cannot, tell the patient why. Keep at arm's length, sit between the patient and the door.

It is impossible to feel confident except with adequate back-up. Do not interview alone but have at least two nurses present and try to do without police. Two nurses are not threatening to an excited person, especially if they are seen as carers rather than authority figures. Large numbers of helpers can be threatening.

Be prepared to listen for 30 minutes or more to a patient's stream of complaints. Appear interested in them and do not give meaningless reassurances or unrealistic promises; interpretations and arguments do not help at this stage. It is always possible to move from contentious areas of conversation to less emotionally charged matters.

Whatever the cause, if violent or disturbed behaviour continues and is threatening it may need to be controlled rapidly. Use haloperidol, 10–20 mg intramuscularly for first injection, repeated every two hours until effective, up to 100 mg in 24 hours, and then changed to 20–40 mg oral dose three times a day (see p. 253). Droperidol can be used similarly in the first two to three days to achieve rapid control; it may also be given intravenously, 5–15 mg, repeated up to four- to six-hourly. Alternatively, use chlorpromazine (100 mg tablet or syrup), two hourly, up to 1 g in 24 hours; an injection must be given deeply intramuscularly and in doses of 50–100 mg, four- to six-hourly. Be aware that this method can cause local pain, acute hypotension or a sterile abscess. The elderly should have lower doses.

If the above doses, even combined, do not calm quickly there is little point in going to higher levels. Consider giving, as well as haloperidol, a benzodiazepine such as diazepam ('Diazemuls') 10–20 mg intramuscularly, two-hourly, up to 80 mg in 24 hours. Midazolam may also be used. Once control is achieved for two to three days, slowly withdraw the benzodiazepine.

The barbiturate, sodium amytal, given intramuscularly as an adjunct to sedative antipsychotics can also be effective for sedation but should not be used for more than a few days (see p. 279). If excitement or aggression persists and repeated injections are required, zuclopenthixol acetate ('Clopixol Acuphase') lasts much longer: 50–150 mg is given by deep intramuscular injection, but should not be repeated for 24 hours. The maximum amount for a course is up to 400 mg total and four injections.

Explain to the patient why and how medication is to be given. Under common law, it can be given in an emergency even without consent. Two or three nurses (either sex, with special training in restraint) working as a team can control and inject a patient without causing injuries. The whole procedure, if carefully done, will not later be resented by the patient. Blood can be taken for analysis at the same time, including for glucose, electrolytes and alcohol.

Rapid, effective control reduces behaviour distressing to patients themselves and results in the possibility of discussion and cooperation in further management.

Drugs used in this way demand close supervision and reassessment every few hours. After such medication, the patient should be nursed lying down, and pulse, blood pressure and respiration monitored.

The search for a firm diagnosis, and the cause, must be pursued as this will decide where to place the patient for further treatment (for hypomania, schizophrenia with aggression, delirium tremens, drug-induced psychosis).

Always check that ancillary investigations have been adequate and complete. Blood and urine analysis for drugs is useful to check for toxic levels, for example: phenytoin, tricyclics, barbiturates, aspirin, in overdoses, and where illicit drugs are suspected – cannabis, amphetamines, codeine, methadone, or morphine. Disturbance apart, patients suffering from toxic effects of drugs (overdose or not) should be treated on medical wards by physicians with expert knowledge. Additional information is available, day and night, from regional poisons information services (see the *British National Formulary* for telephone numbers).

Longer-term management

Acute behavioural disturbance, associated with onset or relapse of a psychotic illness or a drug-induced state, usually settles after a few days with the regime outlined above. During this time the patient may be best managed in a secure, intensive care unit. Continuing with regular neuroleptics at a reduced level may then maintain stability. For a schizophrenic illness, a period of two to three months is often needed to judge the optimum drug dosage, striking a balance between the need to suppress symptoms and yet avoid serious side-effects.

A small group of patients do not improve with high doses of the common neuroleptics and show persistent or intermittent dangerous behaviour for months or years. Acute or long-stay wards are ill-suited to provide care, and 'medium secure units' serve patients with a forensic history. Thus, such patients have been labelled 'difficult to place'. Some districts set up small 'special care' units and others use private specialised units. Such units ideally are secure, provide spacious areas for a range of activities, and allow good observation. Staff are highly trained, with a high ratio per patient, and include a range of disciplines. The multidisciplinary approach reflects the limits of drug therapy and the need for a concerted approach.

A small number of patients have devastating schizophrenic illnesses with active symptoms and serious secondary deficits which have not responded to medication. Here the aim is to prevent deterioration in behaviour and residual abilities while awaiting new, possibly more effective antipsychotics, such as clozapine. The majority of such patients present a complex problem with an interplay of fluctuating psychotic states, mood disturbance, unstable personality, mental impairment or brain damage and drug abuse. This multiple pathology often leads to polypharmacy. Close observation may show a repetitive pattern and identify likely triggers; thus, with foresight, florid episodes may be avoided.

Good practices in prescribing are necessary. For example, minimise use of several drugs of the same class, ensure adequate amounts of an antipsychotic are given (and that the patient is receiving it) before discarding, make only one change in treatment at a time, and give a period of some weeks before coming to a conclusion. Before using a new drug, identify the target symptoms, obtain a base line, and then monitor regularly. In addition to antipsychotics, lithium or carbamazepine may lessen mood changes and impulsive or aggressive behaviour. Zuclopenthixol tablets may reduce aggressive overreaction in mentally impaired or brain-damaged patients. The aim is to suppress distressing symptoms or destructive behaviour with the least amount of drug to achieve this end, that also allows the patient to be alert and mobile. This ensures that input from psychologists, occupational therapists, educationalists and social workers is also effective and forms an integral part of management.

After a violent incident

The incident should be documented and discussed as soon as possible at a meeting of those staff involved, with a view to learning from it rather than to apportion blame. Could the incident have been predicted or averted? Were there warning signs in the patient such as unusual quietness, sullenness, abusiveness or impulsivity? Had the patient been more restless? Were medicines, drugs or alcohol involved? Had there been some provocation? Do any members of staff feel hostile to the patient, and if so are they prepared to discuss this, and does it affect their behaviour? Does the layout of the ward help or worsen the situation? Both tattiness and faulty technology can provoke destructive behaviour.

Plans should be made of how to avoid a further incident, including change in nursing observation and in medication. The hospital should have a written procedure for the prevention and management of violence.

12 Neurotic symptoms and anxiety states

Fears, anxieties, panics, brief bouts of depressive feeling, obsessionality, suspiciousness, irritability, tension headaches, and nausea are experienced on occasion by nearly everyone, usually in a stressful situation or after an event which justifies such feeling as 'normal'. But in some people symptoms occur where the situation does not seem to call for it, or often with greater severity or greater frequency than in the majority. These feelings, which may be termed neurotic, may be associated with sweating, rise in pulse rate, palpitations, indigestion, disturbed breathing, urinary frequency or diarrhoea, all well recognised physical correlates of emotions. These result from arousal in the autonomic nervous system with sympathetic dominance, combined with skeletal muscular tension – the 'fight or flight reaction' of Walter Cannon. Apart from their unpleasantness, which leads the patient to seek relief, they are usually associated with disturbing thoughts and with some disability in free behaviour. The patient is blocked in some way and cannot undertake certain acts in family, social or sexual relationships or in daily work in spite of a wish to do so. A housewife cannot go outside her front door and becomes very anxious if she tries to do so. One man becomes anxious, possibly impotent, in sexual situations. Another starts to get episodes of sudden panic after two of his workmates have died in quick succession. A third, with promotion at work beyond his abilities, gets incapacitating headaches.

In meeting someone with symptoms of this sort, the first question is diagnosis. Is this patient abnormal, oversensitive in the situation and, if so, in what way? Are these symptoms the tip of the iceberg and others will be admitted on questioning? How do they change over time? Is this the reaction of an abnormal personality to stress, or an episode of depressive illness in which depressive mood has not yet appeared but other signs of biological depression are there: early-waking insomnia, loss of appetite, impaired concentration, lack of energy? Is this the beginning of a schizophrenic illness? Anyone over 40 in whom 'neurotic' symptoms are appearing for the first time is probably suffering either from an attack of depressive illness or from some hidden organic disease, possibly a presenile dementia, temporal lobe epilepsy or a carcinoma. Or are we dealing with a person of abnormal personality who, through a sort of emotional colour-blindness, keeps running into social and emotional difficulties and reacting in an upset, angry or depressed way? Occasionally, this seems to be a pattern from a very early age. In some cases, unusual earlier experiences and mistaken learning seem to exert a powerful influence in the present. The patient cannot run away from some current experience, nor face it and act, but remains in inner conflict over what to do. These people may be classified as neurotic or suffering from a personality disorder.

If one identifies what situation provokes the anxiety or other symptoms, one can help the patient to avoid it without shame or, better, it may be possible to change it for him so that it no longer challenges and upsets. But one can also lessen the patient's degree of self-concern, which will have built up on top of the original difficulties. Giving him plenty of interview time conveys that the therapist values him and encourages him to feel better about himself. He learns that he is not alone, that others have troubles like his, that one can talk openly about them and not be criticised or condemned. No guilt or shame attaches to them. He also begins to learn to understand his troubles, not to interpret symptoms as always indicators of physical illness but sometimes of internal emotion or unhelpful reactions to stresses which have become established over the years. In Freud's terms, 'signal anxiety' is indicative of an underlying conflict. The patient sees factors at work which he previously ignored or of which he was unaware. The human mind hungers for explanation and he may need to be given this to explain his own hypersensitivity in terms of a present illness, past mis-education or family dynamics. Patients may also appreciate an account of the disturbed physiology which leads to such distressing somatic symptoms.

Feeling that the therapist understands the patient's case raises hope for the future. Hope may lessen symptoms and milder or less frequent symptoms may allow spontaneous improvement to follow, as illness is not reinforced by more attacks. In some cases, a single hour with the therapist can be enough to start recovery. Suppression of symptoms with a drug may also be helpful. It brings the patient relief, it displays the therapist's power to help, it stops reinforcement of the illness. Except in someone who is using illness to protect himself from something he wants to avoid, removal of symptoms does not result in new complaints but in general benefit.

Psychotherapy of a more advanced kind, whether analytical, cognitive or behavioural, individual or group or family, is an attempt to re-educate the patient, and sometimes his close family too, so that earlier and partly buried misconceptions cease to inhibit or to create conflict. Cognitive therapy can prove very effective in some patients selected on the basis of their personality, cooperation and intelligence.

These methods may be time-consuming and not suitable for everyone; fortunately a good deal can be done in other ways. Counselling and support of a more general kind can help. Drugs may relieve distressing and incapacitating symptoms and allow the patient to be more accessible to a psychological approach. They should not be withheld on some theoretical or moral ground stemming from the belief that psychological problems can only be treated by psychology, or that only the patient's own efforts are valid. The aim must be to spare suffering and increase the person's freedom to act as they wish within the law.

Obviously, where neurotic symptoms are part of depressive illness, schizophrenia or organic disease, medication of the main illness will be important. But where they are localised in a small maladaptive segment of the patient's total behaviour, with very limited symptoms, medication plays a smaller and usually short-term role. Planning a treatment, and expectations from it, must be appropriate to the pattern of illness and distinction made between acute, acute becoming chronic, and the very chronic picture.

Situational

Someone becoming anxious and panicky before an important job interview, a student with worry and insomnia before an exam, a patient awaiting the dentist are examples of acute trouble, where a hypnotic or a daytime sedative, in either case in single dose, may be helpful. The hypnotic must be effective, without hangover, and may need to be repeated for two or three nights at most. The sedative is taken half to one hour before the feared experience, and it is very advisable to try it out beforehand to get the dose and timing right, so that it is neither too strong nor too weak at the time its support is wanted. The person who becomes upset at having to eat in a public restaurant, or to be a passenger in an aeroplane can be helped in the same way, though other treatments may be more curative in the long-run for them.

Short-acting benzodiazepines, such as temazepam (10 mg), thioridazine or chlorpromazine (25–50 mg) by mouth, or a sedative MARI antidepressant are three hypnotics which apply. Although the first is potentially addictive, such very short use is harmless. Bear in mind, though, that stopping a hypnotic often means a poor night or more following, until normality is reasserted. For daytime use, diazepam (2 or 5 or even 10 mg) once only an hour beforehand may be right, and can be repeated only before later stressful events of the same character. Oxazepam (10 or 15 mg) is another alternative, or chlorpromazine (25 mg).

Abnormal reactions to situations can be the result of some frightening incident in the past which may have been forgotten. Abreaction (see Appendix 2) is sometimes helpful in bringing it out. Relaxed by intravenous drug, the patient (in a more suggestible condition) can be induced to talk frankly about relevant emotional experiences and to recall exceptionally potent events. Talking about them into full consciousness may remove their force. Hysterical amnesia and paralysis may be relieved in this way.

Anxiety disorders

The classification of anxiety disorders is less clear than that of the psychoses, and a mixture of different syndromes is common, as well as comorbidity with other problems such as personality disorder and substance misuse.

Pathophysiology

Current neuropharmacological models of anxiety disorders emphasise the role of intact 5-HT pathways from the raphé nuclei in modulating the response to aversive stimuli, and the role of NA pathways from the locus coeruleus in mediating arousal. Panic attacks are viewed as a spontaneous activation of mechanisms close to the respiratory chemoreceptor area which normally mediates the response to suffocation. Panic attacks can be triggered, but only in susceptible individuals, by a range of agents including infusion of lactate or bicarbonate, breathing carbon dioxide, caffeine and cholecystokinin. Theories about post-traumatic stress disorder emphasise the effects of hormones and neuromodulators upon conditioned learning; it is suggested that learning in highly stressful situations becomes over-consolidated and that peptides including adrenocorticotrophic hormone and vasopressin which are known to consolidate memory are opposed by opioid peptides and oxytocin which favour the extinction of conditioned responses.

Simple phobia

The irrational fear and avoidance of specific stimuli such as spiders, cats or dogs, or closed spaces occasionally requires treatment: desensitisation by gradual exposure is the most effective. A benzodiazepine will allow the person to endure closer contact with the feared object whereas a beta-blocker such as propranolol will reduce their tremor and tachycardia but not allow them to make closer contact. Neither of these drugs is useful for this condition in the long term.

Generalised anxiety disorder

Some patients develop free-floating anxiety, not obviously related to any situations, though it often waxes and wanes over periods of weeks. They are tense, irritable, worried, sleep badly, overreact and are jumpy. There may be circadian variations in symptoms, and usually a degree of depression. It may be present on and off at least from adolescence, or it may start in adult life at a time of stress and then continue for a long period. It can be made worse by an environment which cannot be evaded: noise, crowded children in a cramped home, or an unpleasant office where work must go on. Relaxation can be taught, attempts made to clarify the historical origins of the disturbance and durability, and the principles of cognitive–behavioural or interpersonal therapy applied. But it may be humane, or essential, to suppress the symptoms if the patient is to continue at work; psychological methods may fail and other treatment be demanded.

Benzodiazepines are only of use in the short term, for two to four weeks. Thereafter the benefit diminishes and dependence develops, with a rebound exacerbation of anxiety when the drug wears off and a crop of unpleasant withdrawal symptoms if the patient tries to discontinue it. If used, benzodiazepines should be given in the lowest effective dose and on a time schedule which recognises that some of these drugs are metabolised to longer-acting forms. Thus, diazepam has an acute effect over four hours, but a chronic effect due to its metabolites thereafter and this effect may build up slowly, day by day, so that less drug is needed; for example, give diazepam 5 mg, three times a day, and then perhaps 2 mg, three times a day, though it is best not to choose a rigid schedule of this sort but to tailor one to the patient's life. Oxazepam is not metabolised in this way and may, therefore, be preferable.

For longer-term treatment, a monoamine reuptake inhibitor (MARI) or monoamine oxidase inhibitor (MAOI) should be tried in doses similar to those used for depressive illness.

Buspirone is a different class of drug (see p. 276). It has weak anxiolytic properties which develop over two to three weeks. It does not relieve benzodiazepine withdrawal symptoms.

Antipsychotic drugs have little role in the treatment of anxiety but small doses may be used in severe cases resistant to other treatments.

Panic disorder

The term 'panic attack' is often used by patients but is best reserved for sudden episodes of intense anxiety with a feeling of impending disaster accompanied by somatic manifestations of anxiety. These last usually for minutes, occasionally hours. Some patients present to accident centres or to their doctor fearing that they may have a 'heart attack' or other serious illness. Skill is required to convince the patient of the nature of the illness, explaining it in terms of physiological dysfunction. They may be noticed to hyperventilate and need advice about this. Hyperventilation can lead to additional symptoms including paraesthesia and headache, and may also contribute to depersonalisation which is liable to occur.

Patients with panic attacks become afraid of having an attack outdoors or in public where they would feel helpless or self-conscious. This leads to the development of agoraphobia or social phobia. It is then common to experience anticipatory anxiety, similar to panic, when they are called upon to go outdoors or meet people. Behavioural treatments are not always successful. Relaxation techniques and other forms of psychotherapy may be of some help but panic disorder may become chronic.

Beta-blockers are usually ineffective in panic disorder. Although benzodiazepines give some initial relief, this does not endure. With a shorter-acting drug such as lorazepam, the patient develops panic as each tablet wears off and this intensifies their dependence.

Imipramine was the first antidepressant shown to reduce the intensity and frequency of episodes; it is no longer the first choice, but if used it should be started in low doses (25 mg daily) and increased slowly over four weeks to 150–200 mg daily. Other sedative MARIs, for instance amitriptyline or dothiepin, are also useful. More recently it was found that the non-sedative SSRI fluvoxamine was also effective, and this applies also to paroxetine. By contrast, the noradrenaline selective reuptake inhibitor maprotiline does not help.

When using an SSRI the dose should be increased slowly because patients may at first feel more anxious, and may require encouragement to continue the treatment long enough. Monoamine oxidase inhibitors, for instance phenelzine, are also beneficial.

Social phobia

Fear and avoidance of the scrutiny of others may be present from childhood, the patients having for instance been unable to stand or read in class. Situations that they avoid include performing in public, eating in restaurants, or using public toilets. Phenelzine will lessen symptoms in about two-thirds of patients. Start with 10 mg daily, increasing if necessary to 90 mg daily over four weeks. Moclobemide (up to 600 mg daily) is also effective, and better tolerated. The full effect of treatment develops over 16 weeks. If there has been improvement, an attempt should be made to taper off, after six months. In contrast to benzodiazepines, a rebound of the condition will not then occur. Drug treatment should be accompanied by supportive psychotherapy, instructions on self-exposure, or cognitive–behavioural therapy.

Obsessive–compulsive disorder

Obsessional rituals can sometimes be treated with a few hours of behavioural treatment using exposure to the trigger, and response prevention. Some patients are too anxious or distressed to cooperate. In other patients obsessional thoughts dominate the picture. For these groups, drug treatment is often helpful, and clomipramine or the SSRIs are effective whereas the more specific noradrenaline reuptake inhibitor desipramine is not. Doses of fluvoxamine up to 200–300 mg daily, or fluoxetine 20–60 mg daily may be tried. Unfortunately, many patients achieve only a partial improvement; after two months, adjunctive treatment with an antipsychotic drug may be given, for example, sulpiride 200–800 mg daily. Alternatively, a combination of SSRI with lithium may be tried. If there is improvement, treatment should continue for six months and then an attempt to taper it should be commenced.

For those who do not respond to the above, refer to a specialist behavioural unit.

Post-traumatic stress disorder

This condition is recognised as a disabling reaction to a very severe stress, often of a life-threatening kind, which would cause distress in anyone. The symptoms overlap with those of anxiety, depression, simple phobia and obsessive–compulsive disorder. It is important to encourage the patient to talk about and relive the experience (debriefing) soon afterwards. Antidepressants including amitriptyline, imipramine or phenelzine can all be of benefit when continued for eight weeks. The symptoms of anxiety, depression and intrusive thoughts all improve. However, more severe cases seem less responsive. The SSRIs are also of some value, especially for the avoidance symptoms and intrusive thoughts.

Borderline states

A small group of patients, often female, pose a severe problem in diagnosis and management. The condition is usually phasic with periods of relative stability followed by complex patterns of depression, paranoia, behavioural disturbance with injury to self and to others, and abnormal eating continuing for weeks or months. Psychotic-like symptoms may appear temporarily. A variety of diagnostic labels are applied but often as problems persist 'personality disorder' is added. Lithium carbonate or carbamazepine may lessen instability of mood. Low-dose neuroleptics, especially as a depot to ensure adherence, can alter the picture of 'out of control' feelings and behaviour to a more stable state. But such medication must be linked with a consistent and firm overall plan of psychological management.

Chronic illness implies regular reassessment from time to time, measuring relief against target symptoms, and a willingness to rethink treatment. It may need to be altered as people change. Be alert for sudden symptom change, indicating a depressive illness with risk of suicide in one previously with neurotic disability only. Always have a systematic plan of follow-up.

Further reading

CANNON, W. B. (1929) *Bodily Changes in Pain, Hunger, Fear and Death.* New York: Appleton.

MARKS, I. M. (1987) *Fears, Phobias and Rituals.* New York: Oxford University Press.

NUTT, D. & LAWTON, C. (1992) Panic attacks: a neurochemical overview of models and mechanisms. *British Journal of Psychiatry,* **160,** 165–178.

STEIN, G. (1992) Drug treatment of personality disorders. *British Journal of Psychiatry,* **161**, 167–184.

13   Acute and chronic brain syndromes

Acute brain syndrome is also called 'toxic confusional state', 'acute confusion', or 'delirium', depending on its severity. Chronic brain syndrome, most common in the elderly, is also termed 'brain damage' or 'dementia'. Since the chronic syndrome predisposes to attacks of the acute syndrome, both occur most often in old people, although they can occur at any age.

Impairment of memory and other intellectual functions, degrees of disorientation in time and place or even person, partial loss of awareness, perceptual disorders and a general lessening in self-care, with an increased self-centredness, are key signs of brain dysfunction from organic disease. The signs may be mild, moderate, or severe, and may fluctuate from day to day. They may come on gradually and persist, or acutely and be largely or completely reversible. Sometimes an acute attack is superimposed on a chronic illness as yet so mild as to be hardly noticeable.

The two syndromes arise from many physical causes, and every case requires a careful physical examination and appropriate laboratory tests to try to discover the cause. Treatment has three aims: management of the underlying causal condition, if identified; control of symptoms if these are troublesome; and the long-term management of residual symptoms and handicaps.

Acute brain syndrome

Patients with confusional symptoms of recent acute onset often present during treatment for some other condition – medical, surgical or psychiatric – in the home, in casualty, or in hospital. Patients in intensive care or after eye operations are particularly liable to become confused.

If patients are restless, noisy, frightened, aggressive or unable to cooperate in their care, immediate physical treatment may be essential before the definitive cause has been identified. Haloperidol (5–10 mg intramuscularly or intravenously, repeated every two hours), or chlorpromazine (50–100 mg intramuscularly, repeated every four hours with caution) may be required to achieve rapid control. Augmentation with lorazepam (0.5 mg) can be effective. In milder cases, diazepam alone (20 mg intramuscularly or 'Diazemuls' intravenously, four hourly) may be sufficient. For elderly or frail patients, these doses should be halved or less, and intravenous doses should be used only with extreme caution. If less urgent, use oral medication, possibly as syrup. Nursing care of confused patients is important. Nurses must identify themselves positively and make themselves known, by touch as well as voice, each time they do something for the patient.

Delirium caused by alcohol withdrawal is considered on p. 303. A severe delirium caused by antimuscarinic drugs may be relieved by injection of the cholinesterase inhibitor physostigmine (2 mg). The duration of action is about one hour.

After 24 hours it should be possible to reduce the drug dosage and then to stop altogether in two or three days without return of symptoms. Most deliria and other acute syndromes are short-lasting and resolve spontaneously in three to ten days, even without drug treatment, but regular daily assessments are needed. Patients whose acute syndrome takes a quieter path – an episode of partial disorientation and muddle, a sudden unexpected bed-wetting, some strange behaviour, a sudden occurrence of hallucinosis – may best be left without any drug treatment, simply nursed and observed.

When searching for a cause, prescribed drugs should be suspected and stopped if medically possible. In the general medical ward digoxin or pentazocine, for example, may be responsible for an acute brain syndrome. In the psychiatric ward imipramine, amitriptyline, chlorpromazine, antimuscarinic drugs such as benzhexol, lithium and benzodiazepines are examples of commonly used psychotropic drugs which can provoke an acute brain syndrome, sometimes when the dose is excessive and sometimes in the recommended dose recently started.

Individuals vary greatly in their susceptibility to produce toxic blood levels while taking the usual dose. Poor renal performance, for instance, reduces clearance of the drug, and impaired liver function interferes with the removal of the drug and its derivatives by metabolism. Sometimes the delirium may be an inexplicable response to therapeutic blood levels.

In the young, experimentation with euphoriants, illicit drugs or hallucinogenic plants, such as cannabis, khat, or magic mushrooms, may produce delirium and is the most common cause in this age group. Sophisticated urine screening will identify any of these. Dependence on barbiturates or alcohol may cause delirium if the customary drug intake is not kept up, for example following admission to hospital. Patients may not reveal what they feel to be a shameful habit, making the diagnosis that much harder.

Thiamine (B_1) deficiency, arising through alcoholism, malnutrition or excessive vomiting, may present as a confusional state but other neurological signs (nystagmus, double vision, external ocular palsy, ataxia, cerebellar signs and peripheral neuropathy) constitute Wernicke's encephalopathy. This is an emergency requiring thiamine injection to reduce the degree of permanent brain damage and Korsakoff's syndrome.

Serious infection with a fever, even mild infections in the elderly, congestive heart failure, anaemia and renal failure may be physical causes of a brain syndrome. Electroconvulsive therapy (ECT) can lead to confusion for a limited period, especially in elderly patients.

To discover the causal disease may require a search for subdural haematoma, a cerebrovascular accident, an endocrine disturbance, or recognition of an unadmitted drug overdose. When the symptoms of the acute syndrome have cleared and the underlying cause of the attack found, if it is possible to do that, and treated, make sure there is no residual mental deficit. The acute attack may have been made more likely because of a gradually developing chronic brain syndrome which needs attention.

A new cause of delirium is the acquired immune deficiency syndrome (AIDS), because of cerebral effects. The principles outlined are still appropriate for the control of an acute brain syndrome occurring in a patient with AIDS. A complication arises from the danger to staff of infection from an uncooperative patient.

Chronic brain syndrome

The progressive loss of faculties, often behind a facade of politeness and social facility which hides deterioration, must be distinguished from the pseudodementing depression of the elderly. Pseudodementia responds to antidepressant drugs or ECT or, temporarily as with depressive illness, to a night of complete sleep deprivation; chronic brain syndrome is not reversible unless its physical cause is treatable and found early.

The cause of chronic brain syndrome is usually the senile form of cerebral degeneration of the Alzheimer type. Less often the damage is the result of cerebrovascular disease. Other, less common causes include chronic inflammatory conditions or systemic lupus erythematosus, the effects of trauma, transmissible degenerative disorders such as Creutzfeldt–Jakob disease and genetic conditions such as Huntington's chorea. Subdural haematomas, benign cerebral tumours such as meningiomas and possible 'normal pressure hydrocephalus' can be treated successfully.

In practice, an energetic diagnostic search is made only in those patients in whom, by youth or history of rapid onset or distinctive clinical picture, a senile or multi-infarct dementia seems unlikely. To investigate fully every elderly person with a dementing syndrome is not practicable.

Depressive feelings and illnesses

Patients with brain damage sometimes show fluctuating mood swings, anxiety, irritability, or feelings of depression secondary to themselves recognising, if only in part, their disabled state. This lability of mood must not be mistaken for a depressive illness for it does not respond to antidepressant medication or to ECT and may be made much worse if they are used. Agitation may be lessened with small doses of antipsychotics. Patients with recent strokes or other causes of brain damage commonly develop depressive illness. In many cases the symptoms are improved by antidepressants.

Management

The patient with a damaged brain is more sensitive to psychotropic drugs and so requires them in smaller quantities to avoid toxic effects. When a patient is admitted, a wise move is to stop all psychotropic drugs, review the usefulness of the others, and observe if the mental state improves.

Insomnia should first be tackled by general methods before resorting to hypnotics. A regular routine, hot milk at night, avoidance of indigestion, constipation or nocturia by means of a sensible diet, attention to the warmth and weight of the bed-clothes and height of the pillow, and so on, may solve the problem.

Improving the patient's bodily health may have an impressive effect on his mental state and behaviour. Urinary infection, gastrointestinal upset and respiratory infection may need to be treated. More serious medical conditions such as diabetes or cardiac failure may be uncovered by an appropriate medical assessment. However, in spite of such measures, restlessness, especially at night, irritability and insomnia may require drug treatment.

Thioridazine (25–50 mg) or promazine (25 mg twice daily and/or at night) may be effective. There is the risk of anticholinergic side-effects with thioridazine. Small doses of haloperidol may be tried as an alternative, but carry the risk of extrapyramidal side-effects. The generally benign benzodiazepines are less safe. They are potent causes of ataxia and delirium in the elderly and in the past, when still prescribed, barbiturates and bromides caused serious problems. Any psychotropic drug in bigger doses may cause incontinence and falls, even before confusion.

There is no scientific evidence that so-called 'cerebrovascular vasodilators' improve cerebral function. Acetylcholine precursors or cholinesterase inhibitors such as 'Tacrine' have so far not proved worthwhile either. Vitamins should only be prescribed where the patient has had an inadequate diet for some time, has had a gastrectomy or other interference with intestinal function, or has frank symptoms of a vitamin deficiency with laboratory evidence justifying the diagnosis. The long-term management of patients with chronic brain syndrome includes the encouragement of physical independence, and the exercise of the remaining intellectual and social faculties, through provision of suitable activities. Simple tasks can improve the quality of life of patients with dementia, and simple techniques and clear labelling of rooms can increase reality orientation.

Further reading

ADAMS, F. (1988) Emergency intravenous sedation of the delirious medically ill patient. *Journal of Clinical Psychiatry*, **49**, (suppl. 12), 22–26.

LINDESAY, J., MACDONALD, A. & STARKE, T. (1990) *Delirium in the Elderly*. Oxford: Oxford University Press.

14 Extrapyramidal reactions

Extrapyramidal reactions are important side-effects of psychotropic drugs, especially the antipsychotic drugs, and, more rarely, high doses of certain antidepressants or lithium. These neurological side-effects should be recognised by psychiatrists but may not be by clinicians in other specialties. Signs vary from the barely noticeable to the very obvious. Four types of reaction are described: acute dystonia, Parkinsonism, akathisia, which occur early in the course of treatment, and tardive dyskinesia, which develops later on.

Dystonia is a distortion of posture caused by a spasmodic involuntary contraction of one or more muscle groups. Acute dystonia comes on suddenly. It occurs early in the course of drug treatment, sometimes after the first dose, and is more common in young males. Spasm of the muscles of the jaw, neck, spine or eyeball can occur and cause trismus, torticollis, opisthotonos or an oculogyric crisis, depending on the muscle groups affected. The patient may writhe, twist, protrude or bite the tongue, or have difficulty swallowing, breathing or speaking. It is sometimes painful and often frightening. So bizarre are these symptoms that hysteria can mistakenly be diagnosed. The patient may present as an emergency in casualty, or it may be an alarming new symptom in the course of a psychiatric illness.

Akathisia is the name given to a compulsive motor restlessness, especially of the legs, usually accompanied by an unpleasant sense of mental agitation. The name means an inability to sit down, reflected in the term 'the jitters'. The patient with akathisia will stand leaning against a wall, alternately lifting one leg and then the other or, when sitting down, swing or cross and uncross the legs with a greater than usual frequency. The continual activity and apprehension can mislead so that more drug, not less, is prescribed for control. Akathisia is a common reason for patients to discontinue medication themselves.

Parkinsonism resembles post-encephalitic Parkinson's disease in excessive salivation and seborrhoea. Because the cause is a drug effect, the term pseudo-Parkinsonism is sometimes used. Tremor, unusual early on, becomes more common later. Severity varies from the barely perceptible absence of facial expression and stiffness of posture or gait, to complete immobility. Cog-wheel rigidity, especially in the wrists, is a sensitive sign. Drug-induced Parkinsonism is the most frequently encountered of the extrapyramidal reactions. Weeks may elapse between the start of drug treatment and symptom onset. It is more common in older patients and in females. The diagnosis is readily overlooked, the clinical picture being mistaken for apathy or even depression or schizophrenia. This 'akinetic depression' responds to anti-Parkinsonian drugs. Some degree of Parkinsonism may have to be tolerated because of the drug dosage required to maintain control of a psychosis.

Tardive (delayed) dyskinesia occurs with increasing exposure to years of antipsychotic treatment. Involuntary movements of choreiform or athetoid type affect the orofacial and laryngeal muscles. Smacking of the lips, grimacing, tongue protrusion, grunting and blepharospasm are often striking. Less commonly the trunk and limbs are affected, resulting in abnormal posture and gait, sometimes grotesque in severity. Old age, brain damage and female sex appear to predispose to tardive dyskinesia which develops in a persistent form to the extent of about 2.5% of patients per year during long-term treatment. In the elderly, 10% develop this condition within one year of treatment.

Patients who develop Parkinsonism early in treatment are more at risk of later tardive dyskinesia. Cases have been reported in schizophrenics who have not received neuroleptics, presumably resulting from brain pathology.

The range of disordered movements suggests that tardive dyskinesia is not a single entity. The term tardive dystonia describes more severe cases with postural abnormalities and limb movements.

Differential diagnosis

Anxiety, agitation and depression can be excluded with greater certainty if the doctor is aware that the patient either has taken recently, or continues to receive, a drug which can produce extrapyramidal side-effects. Hysteria, encephalitis, Parkinson's disease and Huntington's chorea may be diagnosed in error. Trismus or 'lock-jaw' may suggest tetany, especially if the patient is hyperventilating. Dystonia and tardive dyskinesia might also suggest tetanus but the relaxation between spasms, the relative absence of pain, and the normal movement of other muscles distinguish these drug-induced conditions from tetanus.

If the conditions are mistaken for partly-controlled mental illness there is a danger of antipsychotic drugs being prescribed with a worsening of side-effects. If in doubt about whether the signs are those of mental illness or side-effects, then the effect of an intravenous injection of procyclidine (5–10 mg) should be observed. Alternatively, the drug should be reduced or stopped and the patient observed. Patients should be warned of the possibility of these side-effects before commencing treatment in order to reduce anxiety and avoid a delay in their seeking help.

Pathophysiology

Extrapyramidal side-effects result from the blocking action of antipsychotics at DA receptors in particular areas of the brain, especially the basal ganglia including the corpus striatum. Within the caudate-putamen, DA acts as an inhibitory transmitter on a variety of post-synaptic neurones, especially cholinergic ones. Thus antipsychotics produce a release of acetylcholine, and anticholinergic drugs are needed to relieve acute dystonia, Parkinsonism and, to a lesser extent, akathisia. On the other hand, tardive dyskinesia seems to develop in a way resembling denervation hypersensitivity (see p. 26) during long-term blockade of DA receptors. It can be revealed on reducing antipsychotic medication, and temporarily suppressed by increasing the dose. Anticholinergic drugs worsen it, as do DA agonists such as L-dopa and bromocriptine, and SSRIs.

Interestingly, the occurrence of acute dystonia corresponds to the time of increased release of DA from nigrostriatal neurones, because of blockade of feedback inhibition (see p. 26). During long-term treatment, these DA neurones eventually become quiescent, so that there is less DA released while DA receptors remain blocked. This phenomenon – which does not occur with clozapine – may correspond to the delayed development of Parkinsonism.

Treatment

Acute dystonia can be reversed in 15 minutes or so by procyclidine (5–10 mg given intravenously or intramuscularly) or by benzotropine (1–2 mg), followed by oral procyclidine, orphenadrine, benztropine or benzhexol until control is established.

Akathisia can usually be controlled or lessened with oral anticholinergic drugs. Alternatively, a beta-blocker such as propranolol (20–40 mg daily) may be helpful. Should they fail, then a reduction in dose should be considered. For short-term treatment, a benzodiazepine such as diazepam may be added.

An attempt to control or lessen Parkinsonism by altering dose frequency or reducing the dose of neuroleptic should be considered before prescribing anti-Parkinsonian drugs. For example, 25 mg fluphenazine decanoate every two weeks could be given weekly as 12.5 mg, which reduces the peak levels occurring in the blood soon after the drug is given; or the period between doses may be extended to three to four weeks. Reducing the dose of neuroleptic carries a risk of relapse of mental illness. If Parkinsonian symptoms are distressing, or if they persist after adjustment of the dose, then anticholinergic drugs should be prescribed. Patients should be advised that they can keep the dose to a minimum by adjusting it themselves, but they should not stop anticholinergic drugs abruptly as this leads to transient unpleasant feelings. L-dopa and bromocriptine which are valuable in Parkinson's disease are not useful in drug-induced Parkinsonism.

Tardive dyskinesia can be worsened by anticholinergic drugs but is not caused by them. If early signs appear then anticholinergic medication should, if possible, be reduced, and a reduction of the antipsychotic should also be considered. However, the latter increases the risk of relapse which must be balanced against the disability of the dyskinesia. Frequent review of the need for long-term or high-dose antipsychotic medication is an important part of good practice. For instance, all patients on long-term maintenance treatment should be reviewed at least once a year, and the less stable ones more often. Sulpiride, remoxipride and clozapine may carry less risk of tardive dyskinesia than other antipsychotics. There is no specific treatment for the condition, but in severe cases a switch to clozapine may be justified. Tetrabenazine (75–200 mg daily) may help but, as with an increase in the dose of antipsychotic, the suppression of dyskinesia is usually transient.

When using depot injections, anticholinergic drugs may be needed for only a few days immediately after each injection, especially with fluphenazine decanoate, when serum levels are increased. The patient may be the best judge of need, dose and frequency of anticholinergic. Intramuscular anticholinergics given with the depot injection as an alternative to oral drug gives cover for 24–48 hours.

Routine prescribing of anticholinergic drugs at the commencement of treatment with antipsychotics is undesirable, because not all patients develop extrapyramidal side-effects. However, haloperidol and trifluoperazine are particularly liable to cause dystonia and Parkinsonism, and these should usually be combined with an anticholinergic drug. Higher doses of haloperidol used in mania seem less liable to do so than lower doses. Chlorpromazine and thioridazine which have intrinsic anticholinergic properties are less liable to produce early extrapyramidal side-effects. The newer 'atypical' antipsychotics such as the benzamides – sulpiride and remoxipride – are less liable to produce early extrapyramidal side-effects, probably because they are selective for some types of DA receptors, and are therefore more potent in the limbic areas of the brain than in the basal ganglia. Clozapine and risperidone are also less likely to produce early extrapyramidal side-effects; the reasons are complex and probably include their potent actions on 5-HT-2 receptors, and, in the case of clozapine, on muscarinic receptors with less effect on D-2 receptors in the basal ganglia.

Tolerance to Parkinsonian side-effects of antipsychotics does develop, and then anticholinergic drugs may no longer be required. Their gradual withdrawal, by several dose reductions, should be tried occasionally; sudden withdrawal may provoke more severe Parkinsonism as the nervous system may have developed some physical dependence.

Some patients experience a 'buzz', especially with benzhexol or procyclidine, and develop dependence with a desire for higher doses. Their requests for extra anticholinergic medication should be carefully recorded to avoid double prescribing, and they should not be issued with a prescription unless there is definite evidence that they experience extrapyramidal side-effects.

Further reading

CUNNINGHAM-OWENS, D. G. (1990) Dystonia – a potential pitfall. *British Journal of Psychiatry*, **156**, 620–634.

MARSDEN, C. & JENNER, P. (1980) The pathophysiology of extrapyramidal side effects of neuroleptic drugs. *Psychological Medicine*, **10**, 55–72.

15 Disorders of childhood

Many psychological disturbances are a normal part of development. Transient fears of strangers, animals and imaginary monsters are all appropriate at certain ages; a degree of defiance and recklessness is an expected part of the acquisition of independence. Parents or teachers rather than the child present the complaint; referrals to a clinic may therefore stem from the difficulties of a depressed, obsessional, inexperienced or rejecting adult in coping with an essentially normal child. Assessment must therefore be directed to the child's home and school as well as to the individual child. Whether a child needs treatment is based on an evaluation of the following features:

(a) the duration of symptoms: a short-lived tendency to isolation during a time of stress might wisely be regarded as benign and self-limiting; persistent and prolonged social withdrawal probably means something is wrong

(b) the developmental stage of the child: wetting the bed in a four-year old is probably not an indication for treatment, but if frequent in a ten-year old it very likely is

(c) the number and severity of symptoms: minor rituals and compulsions are unremarkable; but pervasive and severe obsessions causing suffering need treatment

(d) the handicap which the symptoms impose on normal psychological development. This is usually the important consideration and requires an understanding of the major influences for good and ill in a child's life.

Hyperkinetic behaviour in a child from a normal home may disrupt relationships and warrant treatment with stimulant drugs, while for a child in a deprived environment overactivity may be the only way to get adult attention.

The place of drugs

A decision to use drugs as a part of the treatment plan depends on whether the symptoms are likely to be suppressed by a drug, the side-effects of the drug, and the chances of getting the same or better results with psychological treatments alone. Also drug treatment is symptomatic and will not alter fundamental pathological processes.

In general, be slower to prescribe for children than for adults. Nevertheless, serious psychiatric symptoms are such a barrier to normal development that, when psychological or social treatments are ineffective, useful medication must not be withheld for ideological reasons.

Drugs should only be given for definite indications and are uncommon in clinical practice. Drugs should be given as one part of a management programme, supported by careful explanation and by discouragement of any tendency for the child or the parents to place the responsibility for the child's conduct on the drug. Many parents, teachers and social workers react with such suspicion to the introduction of a drug that a sensitive and understanding discussion of its value is required to encourage cooperation and ensure that the child gets what is prescribed.

The effects of psychotropic drugs are not as well known for children as they are for adults. Children metabolise most drugs more rapidly than adults and the dose-response differs from that of adults. The intended action of a drug for a child may differ from the actions expected in adult psychiatry. For these reasons, it is not safe to calculate the child's dose from the adult dose corrected for body weight.

Start the drug in a low dose and then assess the effects of increasing the dose gradually. The most common indications for psychotropic drug prescription are nocturnal enuresis, disorders of sleep, hyperactivity, depression and anxiety, conduct problems in the retarded, and symptoms of childhood psychosis.

Nocturnal enuresis

Most children who wet the bed do not come for treatment. Indeed, bedwetting does not usually get medical intervention before the age of six years, at which age 80% of children are dry. Some children are ashamed of wetting and distressed by their apparent weakness; for others bedwetting is a focus for rejection by exasperated parents.

Nocturnal enuresis is usually simple to treat symptomatically; there need be no hesitation on the grounds that treating a symptom will worsen an underlying psychiatric condition. Rather, abolition of enuresis is likely to improve the child's sense of well-being. Initial assessment should include identifying other problems, and appraising the child's psychological strengths and weaknesses and those of the family. If micturition is normal in the daytime and no abnormality is found on physical examination, neurological investigations need not be done. Urine should be cultured, especially in girls, and any infection investigated and treated.

A record of dry and wet nights is then kept by child and parent in the form of a star chart. Sometimes this is sufficient treatment. The most effective treatment and the safest is the enuresis alarm: the child soon learns to wake and pass urine when the bladder is full. If the alarm fails or is impractical due to family circumstances such as overcrowding, then tricyclic antidepressants in low doses can be tried. Their action is rapid; they usually reduce wetting within a week. Relapse, however, is common when treatment is stopped. Tricyclics can be toxic drugs. They should not be given lightly, nor to exceptionally young children. A special hazard is accidental overdose of the palatable elixir by very young children. If there are young children in the house, precautions must be taken against children, especially other than the patient, taking the medicine themselves. The three-year-old is particularly inquisitive and vulnerable. If drug treatment is to be prolonged then cardiovascular status should be monitored.

If the handicap from the enuresis justifies prescription, then intranasal desmopressin (20–40 mcg) at bedtime is a helpful short-term remedy. Imipramine in a dose of   0.5–1.5 mg/kg is also suitable; if 50 mg given two hours before bed is not effective, there is no point in trying higher doses. Imipramine probably works by an unidentified central effect separate from its antidepressant and peripheral effects. If a tricyclic fails to work, more complex behavioural approaches for teaching continence are available.

Sleep disorders

Simple sleeplessness is often transient, requiring little intervention. The disturbance to parents may be much greater than any to the child. It is usually a better goal that the wakeful child should play quietly in his/her own room than that the usual hours of sleep should be extended by hypnotics. However, when an established sleep rhythm has been disrupted, for example by a period of distress, a short course of an hypnotic drug may be useful.

Short-acting drugs are preferable. Unfortunately, all are likely to exert a sedative action the next morning, and so impair learning ability. Anti-histamines, such as trimeprazine, help sleep but only in the short term. Chloral hydrate in a dose of 40 mg/kg is sometimes effective. Night terrors are to be distinguished from nightmares. In night terrors, the child wakes confused and in a panic from deep sleep and does not remember the episode. Night terrors have no sinister significance but may be associated with other rather benign problems of Stage IV sleep such as sleep-walking. Reassurance for the parents is usually all that is required. When night terrors do cause suffering or handicap, diazepam in a dose of 0.1–0.3 mg/kg will reduce the frequency and diminish the proportion of time spent in Stage IV sleep.

Hyperactivity or attention deficit disorder

Many children are boisterous and energetic and may be described as overactive by harried caretakers; but these are not grounds for formal diagnosis or treatment. The few children who are chaotic and ill-regulated in their behaviour, inattentive to the point where their ability to learn is impaired, need a full psychiatric assessment and possibly treatment. The treatment plan is guided in part by the pattern of behaviour shown, in part by the psychological and physical causes, insofar as these can be known.

If the chief difficulty is defiant, aggressive and unruly conduct, then behaviour modification techniques are likely to be at least as effective as drugs, and are usually best presented in combination with family counselling. If the chief difficulty is in poor academic learning, then remedial education is likely to be the most important intervention, with individual counselling also having a part to play in counteracting the sense of failure which may have arisen.

Medication is most helpful when the chief difficulties are inattentive, disinhibited, disruptive behaviour and poor concentration preventing psychological treatments from working. This is regardless of whether brain damage is the cause. The first choice in drug treatment is a stimulant, preferably methylphenidate in a daily dose of 0.25–1.0 mg/kg body weight. Dexamphetamine and pemoline are alternatives. The drugs lead to an improvement in the behaviour problems, and to better performance on laboratory tests of sustained attention, motor control and reaction time. These are not paradoxical effects, but similar to those seen in normal adults and intelligent children. The effect of methylphenidate is rather short-lived, lasting for a few hours only, and dosage adjustments can therefore be made at short intervals. A starting dose of 5 mg can be doubled after three days and thereafter increased in 5 mg increments to the optimal dose for the individual. Twice- or thrice-daily dosage may be necessary because of the drug's short half-life. The most common unwanted effects are appetite suppression and sleep loss, usually transient and dose-related. Growth retardation can take place with long-term, high-dose medication, possibly due to endocrine changes unrelated to appetite suppression. Methylphenidate can lower the threshold for epileptic seizures; dexamphetamine is therefore preferable for epileptic subjects. Misery and irritability, especially in those with brain injuries, may be another stimulant side-effect. Stimulants, excepting pemoline, are legally controlled substances. Although addiction has not been reported as a consequence of taking prescribed drugs in therapeutic doses, children may find that they are able to sell their tablets illicitly.

The need for careful monitoring of action is all the greater because different psychological processes respond to different doses of drug: concentration often improves at a lower dose than does overactive behaviour. Indeed, a dose which is optimal for restless behaviour may actually lead to deterioration in the ability to attend. Both need to be assessed; the desired goal must be clear. The uncertainties surrounding the use of stimulants are emphasised by the enormous difference in practice between the USA, where more than half a million children receive such drugs, and the UK, where this treatment is given exceptionally. Benzodiazepines should be avoided: they are useless and sometimes harmful. Major tranquillisers can control wildly overactive behaviour when stimulants fail, but this is usually at the price of damaging the ability to learn. Low-dose haloperidol in a dose of 0.02–0.08 mg/kg is preferred. Tricyclic antidepressants, such as imipramine, in low dosage of 1.0 mg/kg have an effect similar in kind to that of the stimulants; but their effect is sometimes transitory and they carry a higher incidence of side-effects, especially cardiovascular ones.

Affective states

Depressive conditions can occur in children before puberty, but presentation can differ from that in adults. In children, aggressive and defiant conduct, decline in school performance, and unexplained pains may indicate depression. The place of antidepressant medication is controversial: trials have failed to show a clear superiority over placebo for either tricyclics or serotonin reuptake inhibitors. Nevertheless, clinical experience suggests that tricyclics can be helpful in those cases with clearly defined depressive syndromes.

A conservative approach is to prescribe antidepressants, say imipramine in a dose of 50–125 mg daily, only when the symptoms of depression as seen in adults are present and psychological treatment has failed or is impractical. Monitoring with electrocardiography (ECG) and blood levels should be undertaken.

Similar medication can be advised for refractory school refusal when depression or pathological separation-anxiety are involved, in combination with family counselling and graded reintroduction to classroom study.

Clomipramine and fluoxetine both have some value in reducing the severity of symptoms in obsessive–compulsive disorders. Non-specific monoamine oxidase inhibitors have little value for children, especially since dietary precautions can be impossible to maintain. Benzodiazepines are seldom effective in reducing anxiety, and carry the hazard of impairing concentration and learning.

A large number of those who present with major depression between the ages of 6 and 12 will develop bipolar disorder before they are 20; follow-up should be provided with this in mind.

Psychosis

The symptoms of infantile autism place a serious handicap upon a child, and are usually rather static. A painstaking and lengthy educational approach has most to offer, and most parents will need support in coping with the difficulties of care. Neuroleptic treatment has a small but definite role in controlling agitation and stereotyped repetitive behaviour, which it can do in relatively low dose, for instance thioridazine 50–100 mg daily.

Bleulerian schizophrenia, occasionally seen in prepubertal children, can be overdiagnosed if one fails to appreciate the frequency in normal childhood of some blurring between fantasy and reality. When hallucinations or delusions are present, then their control with phenothiazines or other neuroleptics follows similar principles to those governing adult treatment. Children seem to be more prone than adults to acute dystonia but less likely to develop Parkinsonian symptoms. Long-term dyskinesias are also reported, although their frequency is unclear.

Conduct disorders in the mentally impaired

The approach to prescribing for the mentally impaired is discussed in the following chapter.

Large doses of neuroleptics sometimes quieten aggression but carry high risks of causing movement disorders, especially in the brain-damaged. Large doses also reduce attention and learning, crucial abilities in all children and especially so in the impaired child. Surveys show that, in spite of these hazards, long-term, high-dose phenothiazines are prescribed for a large proportion of mentally retarded, psychotic children in institutions. This practice is not sound. Behavioural programmes often achieve good results without medication.

However, some handicapped children express their psychoses and mood disorders with altered behaviour: aggression is the most troublesome. Here careful use of antipsychotics, antidepressants, carbamazepine or lithium can further behavioural and social programmes of care.

Paediatric doses

Titration of dose against response is the soundest way of prescribing. The doses recommended here are guides to decide a starting dose based on milligrams per kilogram of body weight. Individual differences in children at each age are so great that weight is a better guide to dose than age. The approximate average weight of a six-year-old child is 20 kg (3st 3lbs), a ten-year-old 30 kg (4st 10lbs), and a 15-year-old 50 kg (7st 12lbs). As adulthood is reached and metabolism slows, the dose per kilogram of some drugs, if used long-term, may need to be reduced.

The following dose/weight schedule is a guide.

Imipramine, 0.5–1.5 mg/kg for enuresis; 1.5–3.5 mg/kg for depression.

Methylphenidate, 0.25–1.0 mg/kg; dexamphetamine, 0.1–0.5 mg/kg; pemoline 0.5–2.0 mg/kg for hyperactivity.

Thioridazine, 1.5–3.5 mg/kg; chlorpromazine, 1.5–3.5 mg/kg for psychoses.

Haloperidol, 0.02–0.08 mg/kg for hyperactivity; 0.1–0.5 mg/kg for control of psychotic symptoms.

16 Mental impairment or learning disability

Impairment of mental development from birth or early years was called mental deficiency, mental handicap or mental retardation. Learning disability, a term introduced by the Department of Health, is now commonly used in Britain for those needing special services, but mental impairment, the term used in the Mental Health Act 1983, though clinically ambiguous, is also in current use.

The mentally impaired are far more likely than other people to suffer from mental illnesses. Some 8–15% have psychoses and half of those in hospitals have neuroses or behavioural disorders such as hyperkinesis, autism, hysteria, and anxiety states, and some 25% have epilepsy. But hospitalised patients reflect a highly selected group and do not indicate a prevalence in the overall population.

These disorders may benefit from drug treatment. Symptoms and signs of mental disorder in such patients are often dissimilar to those of normal intelligence because of the effect of low intellect on use of language. Thus, mental illness is more likely to be expressed as altered or unusual behaviour than in complaints about anxiety, depression, delusions or hallucinations. For this reason, a formulation of the clinical problem in terms of conduct, including the influence of the immediate social environment, is essential. Drugs can then be prescribed for a defined purpose and preferably for a stated period when effectiveness can be reviewed. Avoid long-term prescribing for indeterminate sedation or behavioural problems.

An acutely disturbed person, for instance, may be sedated for a few days as a way of breaking up a fraught situation, with the aim of commencing a programme of social contacts, reassurance and occupation from a calmer baseline. Anxiety may be relieved by daytime sedation, a depressive illness by a tricyclic antidepressant and schizophrenia-like illnesses with long-term neuroleptics. Instability of mood, repeated explosive outbursts, or persistent behavioural disturbance may respond to either lithium carbonate or carbamazepine. Drug treatment should be used as part of a planned programme of behavioural management, psychotherapy perhaps, and environmental manipulation.

Drug response is altered by abnormality or damage to brain structure and hence side-effects may readily appear. Be cautious with dose size until experience with a person has taught what is tolerated. Barbiturates especially may make the handicapped patient irritable and therefore phenobarbitone and primidone are unsuitable as anticonvulsants. Because of limitations of memory and reasoning, the mentally retarded patient may not be able to manage their own medication or report side-effects even after training programmes, especially those living outside of hospital. To get the best out of treatment, everyone – parents, relatives, social workers and nurses – must understand and agree with what is planned.

Drug therapy aimed at specific psychiatric disorder is justified with its efficacy assessed against identified symptoms. Too readily, however, long-term psychotropic drugs are given to suppress behavioural disorder by sedation (confirmed by a lack of diagnosis of a psychiatric illness). This accounts largely for the high proportion of mentally impaired who receive such drugs, especially if living in an institution. Such blanket medication is poor practice; remember, too, that brain-damaged individuals are prone to tardive dyskinesia with long-term neuroleptics. Only use medication in these circumstances for clear and short-term aims. Once a crisis has passed, consider psychological ways of encouraging the patient to develop more adaptive behaviour. That requires skilled staff, applying a plan of treatment with patience and consistency. As with all long-term disabilities, review drug therapy every three to six months, as to its aims and the grounds for continuing it.

(The management of children with conduct disturbance is also discussed in Chapter 15 – Disorders of childhood.)

17   Epilepsy

Most people with epilepsy live stable lives without serious mental symptoms. Of those epileptics seen by psychiatrists, about one in six of the total, in the past, were resident in long-stay hospitals for the mentally ill or mentally impaired or in 'epileptic colonies', but now most of these are in small residential units and many will be living independently. Of those referred, a small proportion are diagnostic problems but most are chronic sufferers from epilepsy who also have to contend with something added: neurotic symptoms, personality difficulties with aggression, a psychosis, or the effects of brain damage and impaired intellect. It is these added conditions, both recent or long-term, which have brought them to psychiatric attention. A different problem is in those with an established psychiatric disorder who suddenly have a fit.

The purpose of this chapter is to assist the psychiatrist to assess and manage the drug treatment of fits.

Diagnosis

Inexplicable episodes of aggression, irritability or other behaviour disturbance, bizarre sensations, panics, amnesias, disorientations, or 'absences' are not necessarily epileptic and may result from psychiatric disorders such as early schizophrenia, neurosis, hysteria or a personality disorder. But there may also be evidence of petit mal or temporal lobe epilepsy. Careful description of the behaviour, including that from a witness, and the abnormal mental experience, possibly a period of observation in hospital, and an electroencephalogram may be required to decide.

Major fits may occur in catatonic schizophrenia, in dementia, as an early or late effect of brain injury, after a leucotomy, in alcoholism and other drug addictions, and as a result of excessive drinking of water.

A fit can result from an MARI antidepressant, phenothiazine or other psychotropic drug. MARIs and many neuroleptics lower fit threshold, predisposing non-epileptic patients to have seizures. Rapid dose reduction of sedative drugs (benzodiazepines or barbiturates, for example) may provoke a fit, especially if the drugs have been taken for a long time. An isolated fit may therefore be a drug or toxic effect and treatment is aimed at the underlying condition.

Epileptic patients well controlled on drugs may have unexpected fits or a change in fit pattern. Occasional failure to take anticonvulsant drugs, or taking drugs which change anticonvulsant drug metabolism, or increased alcohol intake, psychological distress and sleep deprivation may all alter fit threshold. A few epileptics learn how to induce fits and some have 'hysterical' fits. Distinguishing between true and hysterical or simulated fits may be assisted by the serum prolactin which is temporarily increased after a true fit but not after a hysterical one. But many drugs, especially neuroleptics, raise the prolactin level largely, and obscure this test.

Drug treatment

A single fit is not necessarily epilepsy. Never give an anticonvulsant drug after only one fit. Look, first, for a medical or neurological cause or a drug effect – and treat this if it is possible to do so. Only prescribe anticonvulsants when these causes have been excluded, where fits are recurring and the patient is embarrassed or in hazard therepy.

The aim is to stop all fits using one drug and without producing disabling side-effects. In practice this ideal cannot be achieved with everyone, but seizures can be controlled completely in over one-half of treated epileptics with only mild side-effects; and another third have fit frequency or severity diminished.

For generalised tonic–clonic fits, carbamazepine, phenytoin or sodium valproate are the drugs of choice. Carbamazepine is preferred to phenytoin as the latter is sedative, can cause hirsutism, coarsening of the face, and gum hypertrophy. Where these drugs fail, even when two are combined, primidone or phenobarbitone, and newer drugs, for example lamotrigine and vigabatrin, can be tried. Primidone and phenobarbitone are sedative and cause irritability and restlessness. Partial fits should be treated in the same way as generalised seizures. Temporal lobe fits are treated first with carbamazepine but response may be poor and another drug tried or added. Petit mal attacks respond to ethosuximide or sodium valproate or, if these fail, clonazepam. Clonazepam is sedative and can aggravate disorderly behaviour. Atypical absence seizures in secondary generalised epilepsy, and myoclonic epilepsies are difficult to control but the same drugs should be tried, usually starting with sodium valproate.

Commence treatment in the new case with a low dose of the chosen drug. If after a week evidence of response is lacking, increase the dose by small increments every few days until fits cease, early side-effects, especially drowsiness, become intolerable, or measurement of the serum level shows the concentration of drug to be at the top of the therapeutic range. For infrequent fits obviously this assessment takes longer.

If fits still occur with one drug in high dose, add a second, still with the aim of using a single drug in the long-term. Start the second drug in a low dose, increasing the dose in small increments while maintaining the dose of the first. When control is achieved, reduce the dose of the first in small steps with the objective of stopping it. If fits reappear the two drugs will have to be used together.

More than two drugs should not be used. The enemy of therapy is sedation which can be reduced or avoided by using lower doses and less sedative drugs.

Epileptics who continue to have fits in spite of medication may not have the intelligence or the personality to cooperate in treatment. Some may not take their drugs at all and others irregularly. Relatives may know and should be consulted. Serum drug levels are a useful check.

When fits continue to occur and are apparently difficult to control, in spite of apparent optimal medication, review all drugs taken including those prescribed for conditions other than epilepsy. Perhaps the number of drugs or their dose can be reduced with a reduction of side-effects and without increasing fit frequency. Changes must be made slowly, to avoid the risk of temporarily increasing seizure frequency. Sometimes fit frequency may drop after an initial rise if the reduced dosage is maintained.

Avoid combinations of drugs with similar actions, for instance primidone and phenobarbitone. Preparations of tablets or capsules containing more than one anticonvulsant drug (no longer available in Britain) should not be used because separate dose adjustment of the constituents is impossible.

Mental disorder

A chronic and stigmatising disorder such as epilepsy predisposes to episodic irritability and moodiness; failures breed resentment, feelings of inadequacy, and of being at the whim of fate. Patients can become religiose, or excessively suspicious of others, and inflexible in their thoughts and attitudes. Drugs such as chlorpromazine or thioridazine can be used to diminish the more disruptive, irritable, aggressive and paranoid symptoms but lower fit threshold; carbamazepine can be effective here. But psychological support and social help including sheltered workshops are a good approach. Rarely, specialised behavioural units are used.

Neurotic symptoms and depressive illness are not uncommon; drug treatment is along the usual lines but with awareness of which drugs alter fit threshold. Because of the added problem of disability due to epilepsy, treatment must include help on social and interpersonal functioning.

Epileptics may develop schizophrenia. Temporal lobe epilepsy, especially of the left hemisphere, carries a special risk of a paranoid schizophrenic illness. These can be treated with phenothiazines but response is variable. Both neuroleptic and antidepressant drugs may alter anticonvulsant plasma levels.

Longer-term treatment

Epileptics free of fits for three years and without EEG evidence of epileptic activity may try a slow reduction of their anticonvulsant drugs over three months with the aim of stopping them. One in three may be able to do without medication. This should not be tried if a seizure is likely to pose a risk to others, to the patient, or carry a social cost. Avoid sudden withdrawal of drugs because of the risk of precipitating a sharp increase in fit frequency or status epilepticus.

Epilepsy legally precludes driving cars until there has been a fit-free period of two years, or where fits occur only in sleep, and day attacks have not occurred for three years. Epilepsy bars the driving of heavy goods or public service vehicles. The sedation from anticonvulsant drugs may make driving vehicles and operating machinery hazardous, especially if the sufferer also takes alcohol.

Anticonvulsant drugs carry an increased risk of teratogenicity. In spite of this, anticonvulsant drugs will need to be continued during pregnancy because of the risk of fitting to mother and foetus should drugs be stopped. The metabolic changes during pregnancy and lactation may cause a fall in serum levels of drugs. Blood levels should be monitored often and especially in the later stages of pregnancy. Most drugs can be continued during lactation because their concentration in milk is not enough to affect the infant; phenobarbitone and primidone are exceptions, as is diazepam.

Epilepsy in children

The drug treatment of epilepsy in children follows the same principles as for adults. Children and their parents require counselling about epilepsy, the actual fits, and the drugs to control them. Anti-epileptic drugs can interfere with learning and produce irritability and behaviour problems. Plasma levels may show toxic levels which are not clinically apparent in the brain-damaged or intellectually handicapped child.

Treatment of status epilepticus

Consecutive seizures without recovery of consciousness between fits is called status epilepticus. The generalised convulsive form is life-threatening because of respiratory obstruction, hypoxic brain damage or cardiac arrhythmia.

The management of status epilepticus comprises: (a) securing an airway; (b) protecting the patient from self-injury; (c) controlling seizures with drugs.

Diazepam can be given as an intravenous infusion for continuous treatment. The dose of drug required is decided from response, effect being assessed after each 10 mg of injection. When seizures subside the infusion can be stopped, and restarted on recurrence of fits. Diazepam (200–300 mg) may be given during the course of 24 hours depending on weight, health and fit persistence. Respiratory depression and hypotension can occur with large doses, as can thrombophlebitis at the injection site. The latter is lessened by using an emulsion ('Diazemuls').

Clonazepam and chlormethiazole may also be used in this way. Paraldehyde remains a useful drug given in a dose of 5–10 ml deep intramuscularly or rectally as a saline enema (see p. 279). Although its effect lasts longer than that of diazepam it is slower to act, and tissue damage with local necrosis and abscess may occur if injected. Diazepam can be given by rectal infusion ('Stesolid') if an intravenous infusion is impossible.

Seizures must be stopped quickly to minimise the risk of brain damage, and if fits do not lessen in, say, half an hour with diazepam in a generous dose, the aid of an anaesthetist should be sought. More energetic measures can then be employed while pulmonary and cardiac functions are safeguarded. In children, febrile convulsions lasting more than 15 minutes require hospital treatment as an emergency.

18 Alcoholism

People can enjoy alcoholic drinks and may, on occasion, become drunk without being alcoholics. Alcoholism is a form of drug dependence. Physical dependence is recognised when abstinence for any reason results in the appearance of withdrawal symptoms – tremor or shaking, nausea, weakness, irritability, insomnia. Psychological dependence has no simple set of agreed signs, but displays itself as uncontrolled drinking. Different definitions describe alcoholism in terms of the distress expressed or observed, the damage to physical health, the difficulty in cutting down or giving up drinking altogether, or the damaging effects to working, social or family life.

Alcoholic patients come to psychiatric notice for three reasons: withdrawal symptoms; referral for the treatment of alcoholism; and longer-term effects, such as brain damage or psychoses. Withdrawal symptoms or even delirium tremens may begin at home, after admission for a non-alcoholic reason to a medical, surgical or psychiatric ward, or after remand in custody – situations where supply of drink is removed. Out-patient referral for treatment of alcoholism is usually on the urging of other people because of the social effects of continuing addiction on the alcoholic or on other people.

Drugs play an important part in detoxification and the treatment of delirium tremens, but they play only a small part in preserving abstinence from further drinking, where management is largely psychotherapeutic and social. Long-term damage causing Korsakoff's syndrome is not relieved by specific drugs but Wernicke's encephalopathy requires urgent medical treatment with thiamine (see p. 131 & p. 313). A few alcoholics develop a schizophreniform psychosis which may respond to antipsychotics.

Attempts to decriminalise drunkenness have resulted in detoxification centres being opened by voluntary organisations. Management is in the hands of staff specially experienced in treating detoxification, with medical care supplied by general practitioners, and in liaison with a hospital physician.

Detoxification and drug treatment

Withdrawal symptoms may be slight or lead to epileptic fits or full-blown delirium tremens. Management often requires hospital admission, especially for the severely affected where there is a risk of death. The principal psychiatric symptoms are insomnia, tremor, weakness, nausea, irritability, confusion, tactile, visual and auditory hallucinations, and terror. Withdrawal fits are common. Acute circulatory collapse, hypothermia and infection may occur and require urgent action. The patient may be dehydrated and hypoglycaemic.

The aim of treatment is the control of psychological symptoms, the prevention of fits and the care of the patient's physical health. Make sure the patient has no secret supply of alcohol or sedative drugs. Experienced physical nursing and close medical supervision are needed. Temperature, pulse and blood pressure must be noted four-hourly and fluid balance recorded. Serum electrolytes and blood glucose need to be checked.

Suppression of psychological symptoms (and prevention of withdrawal fits) can be accomplished with chlordiazepoxide, diazepam or chlormethiazole, the dose depending on age, weight and severity of symptoms: 1 g chlormethiazole (every six hours), or 20–40 mg chlordiazepoxide or diazepam (every six hours) are guide doses. Chlorpromazine or thioridazine (200–300 mg daily) can also be used where disturbance is severe. When symptoms start to wane, these drugs should be steadily reduced to zero over three to seven days, depending on response. Because heavy drinkers have a poor diet, a course of intramuscular vitamins should be given.

The sedative drugs used to control symptoms must be reduced and then stopped as soon as withdrawal symptoms are over, because diazepam, chlordiazepoxide and chlormethiazole are, like alcohol, drugs of dependency to the susceptible and should not be used for chronic treatment. Chlormethiazole should not be prescribed to patients who are still drinking; the combination can lead to fatal respiratory depression. It should be administered to out-patients only under close daily monitoring.

With the exception of disulfiram, no drugs seem to help in the prevention of relapse, although some patients with chronic depressive features do well with lithium or a tricyclic if they take them regularly.

Assess physical health, looking for malnutrition, infections, and peripheral neuritis, and check liver function and test for any signs of an early dementia. Formal psychological memory testing will provide a baseline for the future, and computerised tomography or magnetic resonance imaging indicate degree of brain shrinkage and ventricular dilatation.

Any psychiatric illness must be treated, for instance depression, mania, or anxiety state. Alcoholic hallucinosis or paranoid psychoses respond like schizophrenia to antipsychotic drugs. Stop all alcohol and give the antipsychotic in suppressive doses. The psychotic state usually clears in a few days. Cautiously reduce the dose and stop altogether if symptoms do not recur. About 10% of patients do not remit and require long-term treatment.

Although alcoholism, in itself, does not provide grounds for compulsory hospital admission under the Mental Health Act 1983, such action can be appropriate when delirium tremens or a florid psychosis is present.

Prevention of drinking

If detoxification is needed for the heavily dependent, psychological help begins as soon as the person is accessible. Residential units run by voluntary groups provide care and support for many months to serious problem drinkers to establish abstinence, a process of self-awareness, re-education and peer support. For the less urgent and severe, most districts have set up alcohol advisory centres open to referrals from any agency or to individuals themselves. Thus, excessive drinking can be picked up early (by general practitioners, accident and emergency screening, out-patients, family and friends) and help offered before the pattern becomes entrenched. Centres provide a range of information including contacts for support, Alcoholics Anonymous (AA), and other self-help groups. These provide the basis for long-term management.

For any treatment to be successful, alcoholics have to admit to themselves that alcohol is getting the better of them. They must want to regain self-control. They can be helped by recognition of the situations which particularly provoke drinking and by understanding their own self-condemnation and self-punishment. Some people live in particularly predisposing situations, for example a job which favours a bar life. Social or sexual timidity may be relieved by alcohol. Lack of leisure interests, loneliness at home, or bereavement may lead to drinking. Identification of the pattern and of provoking factors may lead to helpful changes in lifestyle. For most sufferers, complete abstinence from alcohol in any form must be the target; for a few, very limited, moderate drinking may be achievable. Regular contacts over a lengthy period with a doctor, nurse, psychologist or counsellor who will be accepting, encouraging and non-judgemental are likely to aid the patient in achieving rehabilitation. Short admissions to hospital at difficult times can be useful in preventing relapses, but most longer-term treatment is now outside hospital.

Apart from solving the problem of homelessness, a hostel may give valuable support and produce change. Much social help over finance, employment, marriage, loneliness and isolation, and development of new interests may be needed. Special attention must be given to the family. The therapist must be prepared for long-term supervision, for repeated setbacks in some cases, but must never lose heart. Considerable benefit can be expected in two-thirds of cases. The support of fellow sufferers in therapeutic groups can be crucial. One marginally useful method of treatment does involve drugs. The patient, who must be in good health, takes disulfiram ('Antabuse') regularly every morning, possibly under some supervision, for a long period. The drug stops the metabolism of alcohol at the stage of acetaldehyde. Acetaldehyde is a toxic substance producing unpleasant feelings of violent throbbing in the head, dyspnoea, sickness and, in excess, giddiness, failing vision, cardiac irregularity and collapse. The patient on disulfiram learns in hospital that one glass of his favourite drink will provoke unpleasant symptoms, and is thereby helped to avoid the temptation of a single drink when outside (see p. 297). However, this only works if the drug is kept up regularly, and is hazardous in poorly motivated patients. It is also claimed that lithium carbonate if taken regularly may help abstinence, even in the absence of depression.

19 Drug dependence

Dependence on drugs can be divided broadly into psychological and physical dependence. Both have neurochemical counterparts, which differ from one drug to another. For instance, psychological dependence may be mediated by the interaction of drugs including opiates and amphetamines with the mesolimbic dopamine pathway subserving drive-orientated behaviour; craving becomes strongly cued to environmental triggers. Physical withdrawal symptoms from opiates arise in part from disinhibition of noradrenaline neurones in the locus coeruleus (see p. 30), and of other neurones peripherally, including cholinergic neurones in the gut.

Unstable opiate addicts

The more serious problems presenting to casualty, medical and psychiatric services arise in the unstable opiate addicts. These are usually young, immature, often with serious difficulties in maintaining relationships and work, and consequently with formidable social problems. Their addiction history is of switching from one drug to another, whichever is available, and increasing the amounts taken until they have to support an expensive daily habit, all of which aggravates any conflict with the law. The young addict may have dabbled with many drugs, having begun with the less toxic. Later he experiments with opiates, for example heroin or methadone. He begins by taking the drug orally, or by inhalation, and later learns to use intravenous injections. Veins become thrombosed, and a source of systemic infection. When other veins are occluded he may then resort to injecting into the femoral vein. Stimulants and barbiturates are sometimes added to enhance the effect, increasing the risk of fatal outcome.

A drug subculture might provide a reasonably stable and satisfying lifestyle but, even so, there may be accidental or deliberate overdoses, intoxication, infection, including with the human immune deficiency virus (HIV), abstinence symptoms, acute toxic states and social problems such as domestic crises, homelessness, unemployment, and conflict with the law. Illicit drug-taking is usually one symptom of a disturbed personality. A healthy scepticism in the face of an apparent sudden desire to cease drug-taking may be appropriate. There may be new pressures, such as court proceedings or threats of separation from relatives. These are opportunities when the patient is motivated to make important changes, but they may be half-hearted; the drug may be the only aid the patient now has to maintain a semblance of feeling normal. Nevertheless, it may be possible for a case worker to increase the patient's motivation. With encouragement and practical help, the patient may gain in confidence. Such opportunities to promote change should be taken, and the patient should be put in contact with the relevant services.

Principles of management

Drug users should have rapid access to treatment for drug dependence. The stabilisation, withdrawal and long-term treatment of the drug user are the responsibility of the psychiatrist. Addicts who present themselves unexpectedly at hospital may be concerned to get more drugs, so their stories are unreliable. On the other hand they may be suffering from the unwanted effects of serious addiction, especially infections, which must be looked for and treated.

Opiates

The ultimate aim should be total abstinence but, while this is being achieved, 'harm minimisation', particularly in relation to injectable drugs and the risk of HIV infection, is important. This means that information on safer injecting and HIV risk-reduction strategies should be provided, along with clean syringes and needles, to those who continue illicit intravenous use; needle and syringe exchanges exist in many places where there are large numbers of addicts.

Opiates should only be prescribed to out-patients when reasonable steps have been taken to establish that they have a daily habit. Only one person should provide a prescription for a drug of dependence for an individual addict, and the dose should be kept to the minimum required. Prescriptions range from 25–80 mg methadone daily, depending on the length of drug history and the extent of recent drug use.

The organisation of services is based upon collaboration between hospital, general practice and voluntary agencies. Each health district should have a drugs advisory committee with multidisciplinary representation. Most districts now have a community drug team which is usually street-based and works closely with general practitioners, with some advice from a specialist psychiatrist. More specialist care is available for out-patients from drug dependence units, of which there are at least one in each health region. Most clinics aim to provide services for those in a defined catchment area, and are likely to require proof of residence. However, there is also the need to provide services for homeless drug users.

All doctors can prescribe drugs, such as methadone, for addicts; those who do so regularly can apply for a handwriting dispensation (see below). All doctors can prescribe heroin for the relief of severe pain in addicts. Heroin, cocaine and dipipanone can otherwise only be prescribed to addicts by doctors who hold a special licence from the Home Secretary. Licences are usually only granted to doctors working in National Health Service drug-treatment centres.

If a doctor sees a patient who is drug dependent, he must notify the Home Office using a special form. The Home Office keeps an index of addicts which is available to doctors, enabling them to trace earlier contacts made by the individual with doctors.

Patients seeking help because of opiate addiction may have found their lives dominated by the strength of their drug habit. The main steps in the medical management are assessment, stabilisation, withrawal (detoxification) and drug-free rehabilitation.

A patient presenting for the first time for instance in casualty should not be given a prescription for an opiate, but should be referred to the local drugs service for assessment and treatment. However, if a patient is admitted to hospital or detained in a police cell, then assessment and treatment should be carried out.

Assessment

Establish the reasons for which they are seeking help, the recent pattern of drug use, and the history of substance abuse. Do they have a problem with alcohol, benzodiazepines or other substances in addition to opiates? Many use cannabis. Ask about the social situation, any legal problems, and their finances. How much are they spending on drugs? How do they obtain them and is a doctor already prescribing? Try to determine whether they are dependent, by their description of withdrawal symptoms for the various drug groups. Is there any history to suggest underlying mental illness or drug-induced psychosis? Look for current withdrawal symptoms: sweating, running nose and eyes, pilo-erection, abdominal cramps, vomiting, diarrhoea, arousal and restlessness. Examine the pupils which are tiny after opiates and dilated after stimulant drugs; the conjunctivae may be reddened by cannabis. Check the pulse and blood pressure which may be raised by stimulants and by opiate withdrawal. If they are irritable or hostile, they may be intoxicated with alcohol; if paranoid, suspect stimulant abuse, amphetamine or cocaine. Examine the upper limbs for needle marks and thrombosed veins. If in doubt examine also the lower limbs and groin.

A specimen of urine should be taken for analysis. This may confirm the patient's account of what they are using, identify additional drugs which they have denied or not mentioned, or may contradict the patient's claim to be using a drug regularly. If they have a daily habit, then every specimen should contain the relevant drug unless they are obviously withdrawing at the time it is given. It is usual to require two to three specimens of urine provided on separate days to be positive for the opiate, before a prescription is issued for substitution therapy with oral methadone.

Stabilisation

Once it has been established that they are dependent upon opiates, a prescription can be agreed for oral substitution with methadone. The intention is to provide them with a secure supply of an opiate in a less harmful form so that it is not necessary for them to inject themselves or to break the law to obtain drugs. In the medium term, the aim over three to six months is to reduce the dose of methadone gradually and wean them off it.

Treatment should be planned in the form of a contract between the doctor or clinic and the patient. The details will vary depending on the patient, the clinic's facilities and the approach, which should be consistent for all addicts. Having agreed the starting dose of methadone, the prescription will be written for a named pharmacist identified by the patient and contacted by the clinic.

The pharmacist will supply the drug daily but will not supply more drugs or replace them if they are 'lost'. The patient is then seen every week or so for counselling and for support, and encouraged to reduce the dose of the drug. Further urine tests are used, to confirm that they are taking the drug prescribed and no others. The contract will include conditions about the plan for reducing the dose and the total length of treatment which may range from three to six months, and will require the patient to attend regularly and to provide urine specimens on request. The consequence of a patient breaking the contract may be that the patient's course of treatment is temporarily suspended.

The bulk of treatment evaluation suggests that the greatest amount of health gain can be achieved by oral methadone prescribing. Most clinics do not find it necessary to prescribe more than 60–80 mg of methadone daily, or to issue prescriptions for injectable drugs other than to a small number of addicts who have been receiving such prescriptions since the 1970s when that approach was used. For some patients, single daily doses are less helpful than divided doses, because withdrawal symptoms emerge before the next dose is due in 24 hours.

During the period of stabilisation, the patient's use of alcohol and tranquillisers should also be addressed. Ideally there should be a policy about prescribing benzodiazepines to addicts, agreed between the drug services and local general practitioners, to ensure that patients receive prescriptions from only one doctor, and that benzodiazepines are not prescribed other than for patients with confirmed dependence who are receiving counselling to withdraw from them.

Patients who have been using large quantities of drugs or combinations with alcohol and benzodiazepines may need to be admitted for stabilisation. During the admission they are given a prescription for methadone up to 80 mg daily, and alcohol or benzodiazepine withdrawal symptoms are treated.

Detoxification

Many patients find it possible to gradually reduce their dependence on methadone over the course of three to six months and discontinue it. Others find each step in the reduction difficult and are liable to supplement the prescription with illicit drugs, including heroin, which are then detected in the urine. If the patient is unable to reduce as an out-patient, or wants to discontinue methadone more quickly, then in-patient detoxification should be arranged. This may be done by stepwise reduction of methadone at the rate of 5–10 mg a day over the course of 10 days as an in-patient on a psychiatric ward. This may be unsuccessful because patients experience withdrawal symptoms lasting weeks, and their interactions with other patients and the staff can be difficult to manage. An alternative method of detoxification can be used in which the withdrawal is speeded up by the use of naltrexone. However, it must be explained to the patient that this is an unpleasant procedure, and they must be motivated to take part voluntarily.

The patient is admitted to hospital and observed for 24 hours without drugs. Treatment of the withdrawal symptoms is started with lofexidine or clonidine to make sure that these are tolerated (see p. 300). If they are, and if the withdrawal symptoms are not severe, then oral naltrexone is given, leading to the development of acute withdrawal symptoms. These are of maximum intensity at the start, but decline in severity over the course of two to three days. During this time the patient is treated with further doses of lofexidine or clonidine, is under expert nursing observation, and is given much reassurance. They should be able to leave hospital, no longer experiencing withdrawal symptoms, about six days after admission. This regime can be successful on a general psychiatric ward if the staff are familiar with it and have a bed reserved for the purpose. Special care is also required with those who have alcohol problems, which should be dealt with before the opiate detoxification. Patients with grossly antisocial personalities may not be suitable, especially if they are HIV positive.

When clonidine is used, the blood pressure should be monitored and the dose adjusted accordingly. More problematic addicts need longer periods of in-patient treatment which is best provided by specialist units.

Rehabilitation

One of the great challenges for services is to maintain abstinence after it has been achieved. Detoxification is only the first step in a period of rehabilitation. Here, voluntary agencies play a very large part, especially if the patient is sensitive to environmental cues and factors which produce craving and a ready supply. Placement (voluntarily) in a different setting and away from sources of supply, possibly for a year, may be a necessary step. Residential facilities ranging from the Minnesota Model, to Concept House or Christian Therapeutic Communities are of considerable help to many people. Self-help groups run by Narcotics Anonymous operate along the same lines as Alcoholics Anonymous. Individual, family and group psychotherapy may be needed, and for some patients attendance at a day centre is helpful.

Barbiturates

Barbiturates are sedative and anticonvulsant. They are seldom prescribed nowadays following a voluntary agreement among general practitioners not to do so 20 years ago. Their use was associated with tolerance and physical dependence. Overdoses produced respiratory and cardiovascular depression, and death. A dangerous feature was that patients would take their night-time dose repeatedly, after becoming drowsy and forgetting that they had already taken it. Withdrawal is associated with anxiety, insomnia, tremor, convulsions and a confusional state, and other symptoms similar to alcohol withdrawal. A small number of addicts still obtain barbiturates. Withdrawal from them can be managed by switching to chlormethiazole and reducing the dose as in the treatment of alcoholism; the adjustment may take longer, for instance three to six weeks. Irritability and sleeplessness may continue for up to three months: the patient should be warned of this and encouraged to tolerate it rather than seek relief with other drugs.

Stimulants

Amphetamines are no longer widely available on prescription because of a voluntary ban on their use other than for narcolepsy. A few 'diet clinics' prescribe these drugs although there is no medical justification for doing so. Patients become psychologically dependent and ask for private prescriptions for drugs such as 'Tenuate Dospan', claiming to want help to reduce weight. However, amphetamines are easily synthesised and readily available from illicit sources. Their use in small doses produces symptoms of elation, racing thoughts, pressure of speech and overactivity resembling mania but of short duration. Appetite, however, is suppressed. Larger doses produce paranoid symptoms and a state resembling paranoid schizophrenia. This requires hospital admission and can usually be suppressed with haloperidol or chlorpromazine. Sometimes a longer episode of mania is precipitated in a bipolar patient, and schizophrenia may be exacerbated.

The abstinence or crash syndrome results in lethargy, dullness and depression; psychological support may be required for a short period and occasionally antidepressant treatment is needed. There is no medical justification for prescribing amphetamines to addicts; attempts to do so exacerbate the problems of paranoid psychosis, disinhibited behaviour and manic states.

Cocaine produces mental changes similar to those of amphetamines. When used as the free-base ('Crack'), its onset when inhaled is similar to intravenous use, and it is more dependence-inducing. Possible treatments include imipramine and other antidepressants.

Some amphetamine derivatives are metabolised in the body to produce neurotoxic compounds. These can damage particular neurones in animals. It is suspected that 'Ecstacy' (methylenedioxymethamphetamine, MDMA) or its metabolites may damage serotonin neurones causing persistent neuro-psychiatric problems. Parkinson's disease can also result from neurotoxic effects of drug metabolites (see p. 217).

Psychotomimetics

Lysergic acid diethylamide (LSD25) is now prescribed rarely but is used illicitly to enlarge perceptual experience. Emergency treatment may be required during a so-called 'bad trip', which may cause acute distress or result in the person harming himself or others while under the influence of delusions. Management by friends is usually sufficient, but sometimes it is necessary to terminate the acute psychosis, in which case chlorpromazine (50–100 mg intramuscularly) or diazepam (10–20 mg intravenously) are effective. Sometimes the experience is vividly relived later in the so-called 'flash-back' associated with bouts of anxiety and derealisation. Drugs are rarely needed unless the 'flash-backs' are severe, or frequent. Phenothiazines, in small amounts, given for a few weeks or months may help. More rarely, a chronic paranoid psychosis resembling schizophrenia occurs, and should be treated with phenothiazines. This may be a schizophrenic illness which could have occurred anyway. There are no abstinence phenomena.

Cannabis (marijuana) can in large quantities produce a short-lived schizophrenia-like state. It can also, even in small quantities, cause relapses or exacerbations of paranoid psychosis, schizophrenia and mania. These require antipsychotic medication.

Phencyclidine (PCP) ('angel dust') has stimulant and psychotomimetic properties and produces a paranoid hallucinatory state with some features of acute schizophrenia but with more cognitive impairment, visual hallucinations and hyperactivity. One mechanism of its action is blockade of a type of glutamate receptor. It also blocks potassium channels, prolonging action potentials. The psychosis is not easily treated with conventional antipsychotic drugs, but requires sedatives. Fortunately its use in Britain is rare.

There are other substances with an industrial or household use which are sniffed, for example glue, paint thinners, lacquers, some solvents, aerosols and petrol fumes. They are not dangerous in small amounts but rapidly give a feeling of intoxication which may be accompanied by aggressive behaviour and hallucinations. In large amounts or chronic use they are very dangerous, producing cerebellar and renal damage.

Inhalation of volatile substances results in a considerable number of deaths each year and it appears that many who die have been involved in experimental or infrequent use. Professional people with access can become addicted in a similar way to ether, nitrous oxide, cyclopropane, trichlorethylene and other anaesthetic gases. The chronic abuser poses problems similar to those seen with the other addiction groups, in whom lack of motivation to stop is the most serious.

The drug scene

Stimulants and psychotomimetics are used occasionally and unofficially for their mental effects, especially by the young who are interested in the experiences they induce. Only a few people continue taking such drugs regularly and even fewer become addicted, in contrast to alcohol and tobacco. Those who do may suffer from personality problems and it is this group who present to the psychiatrist. The non-medical use of drugs depends on availability and prevailing popular knowledge of their effects. Some can be obtained over the counter: cough mixtures containing morphine or ephedrine, antihistamine mixtures with codeine, for instance.

Legal aspects and notification

The Misuse of Drugs Act 1971 was the first step to provide better control over misuse of drugs of all kinds and laid down rules for supply and possession. 'Controlled drugs' are classified in three grades, depending on harmfulness when abused. Penalties for offences are graded similarly.

Class A: examples – cocaine, diamorphine (heroin), dipipanone, LSD, methadone, morphine, opium, pethidine, phencyclidine and class B drugs when injected.

Class B: examples – oral amphetamines, barbiturates, cannabis, codeine, glutethimide, pentazocine, phenmetrazine.

Class C: examples – meprobamate, certain drugs related to amphetamines such as benzphetamine or pemoline, and most benzodiazepines.

Further regulations (1973) require details about addicts to be notified to the Home Office. The relevant drugs are cocaine, dextromoramide ('Palfium'), diamorphine (heroin), dipipanone ('Diconal'), hydrocodone ('Dimotane DC'), hydromorphone, levorphanol ('Dromoran'), methadone ('Physeptone'), morphine, opium, oxycodone, pethidine, phenazocine ('Narphen') and piritramide ('Dipidolor'). If the treating doctor suspects the patient is an addict, that is, is persistently dependent on the drug, he must notify the Chief Medical Officer, Home Office Drugs Branch, Queen Anne's Gate, London SW1H 9AT, within seven days. If the patient is still being treated a year later, a further notification is required. Details have been limited to personal ones and the addictive drug. Since 1990, a new system operates with more detailed clinical information. This, with personal details, goes, as before, to the Home Office and a copy, without personal identification, goes to local district and regional drug misuse databases. This will provide data on clients, the use of facilities and a guide to future planning.

The Home Office keeps an index of notified addicts and this is available, on a confidential basis, to doctors. Hence it is wise, when faced by a new addict, to check with the Home Office that the addict is not already being treated elsewhere. Write to the Chief Medical Officer or, more simply, telephone 071-273 2213. The response will be by a return telephone call to ensure the caller is a genuine doctor.

The above applies to England, Scotland and Wales. In Northern Ireland, notification is to the Chief Medical Officer, Ministry of Health & Social Services, Dundonald House, Belfast, BT4 3SF, and telephone enquiries to 0232-63939 ext. 2867.

Special prescription pads, FP10 (HP)(ad) are used in hospital to request chemists to issue drugs on a daily basis. Similar prescriptions FP10 (MDA) are for the use of general practitioners to prescribe for daily dispensation.

Special conditions apply to writing a prescription for controlled drugs. It is to be written in the prescriber's own handwriting, in ink, and include the name and address of the patient, the form and strength of the preparation, the dose, the total quantity of the drug, in words and figures, and be signed and dated. Exemption from the handwriting requirement can be obtained for doctors working with large numbers of drug users.

More advice on the Act and Regulations can be sought from the Regional Senior Inspectors of the Home Office Drugs Branch:

London and South-East England	071-273 3530
Midlands, South-West England and Wales	0272-276736
Northern England and Scotland	0274-727149

20   Sexual disorders

Complaints of sexual dysfunction may occur as the presenting feature of a psychiatric illness, or in the course of psychotropic drug treatment, in the setting of a personality problem, or sometimes as a separate source of worry with a request for explanation and reassurance. Some apparently unexplained sexual problems are referred from medical or surgical colleagues because sexual disorders may be considered the psychiatrist's province.

Sexual dysfunction occurs in nearly all psychiatric illness. Depression lowers sexual drive and performance, leading to indifference, impotence or frigidity. In a previously well-adjusted couple, a serious misunderstanding can result. Explanation of the biological nature of the change, and reassurance that normal sexual response will return on recovery from depression, usually enables a couple to accept the situation.

Mania, in contrast, heightens sexual drive and sexual enjoyment. Increased sexual demand in marriage may become a problem for the spouse of a manic patient, and so may promiscuity or sexual deviations as a result of disinhibition. Explanation and reassurance to the well partner assists adjustment but this needs to be long-term with other forms of help for the condition.

Schizophrenia is associated with low sexual drive which, with deficits in emotional display, limit sexual activity. In early onset, marriage is infrequent and fertility is low, especially in males. Sexually embarrassing or deviant behaviour occurs sometimes in chronic schizophrenia and presents potential problems for the community, requiring well planned aftercare. A dangerous condition is morbid jealousy, with paranoia, and often linked to sexual impotence or inadequacy. Lack of sexual experience and poorly controlled impulses in the mentally impaired can lead to deviant or inappropriate behaviour. Recognition of the problems and guidance by a therapist should be of help.

Dementia causes serious problems if disinhibited, embarrassing or unlawful sexual acts occur. Exposure or other indecency may be the presenting feature, almost exclusively in males.

Alcohol abuse results in loss of sexual drive and ability, as does other substance abuse, but can lead to disinhibition.

Sexual dysfunction arising in these ways usually needs no treatment other than of the primary psychiatric illness. Embarrassing or potentially criminal sexual conduct occurring in schizophrenia or mental handicap when related to high sexual drive may respond to drugs which reduce such drive.

The drugs used to treat psychiatric illness often affect sexual function in an unwanted way. Any drug with sedative effect, including benzodiazepines, especially when used in excess, can reduce sexual interest and drive. Neuroleptics and antidepressants can cause impotence, delay ejaculation, or inhibit it entirely. Clomipramine and SSRIs are especially prone to do so, and cause anorgasmia in women. Conversely, they, rarely, produce spontaneous orgasm in women. When tolerance to the drug develops, or the drug is stopped, sexual function usually returns to normal. Many drugs used in general medicine, and which the older psychiatric patient may be taking, also affect sexual function: thiazides, for instance, can cause impotence. Hence the importance of a full drug history.

Sexual dysfunction presenting in the absence of any causal illness requires treatment of sexual performance itself. Sexual problems comprise an increasing part of psychiatric practice because people expect sexual intercourse to be enjoyable and are prepared to do something if it is not. The treatment of primary dysfunction uses a behavioural approach directed to improving the sexual response of a couple to each other. Success depends on motivated, cooperative, sexual partners and a therapist with special skills. Drugs have usually no part in this treatment. Sedative drugs, however, may have a small part to play when anxiety and impotence are linked, especially in the uncertain young man or the overconsciously ageing one. If taken shortly before intercourse, sedative drugs can sometimes improve performance. Drugs are not generally useful for treating premature ejaculation. In women, dyspareunia, vaginismus and anorgasmia are common complaints leading to worry, resentment and a poor married relationship. Drugs are ineffective and may do harm. A behavioural approach is recommended for all these conditions, and is best done by specialist clinics with skilled therapists.

A high level of sexual activity, especially if associated with psychopathic personality or sexual deviance, can be a serious problem in men and may result in crime and loss of liberty. Drugs which reduce sexual drive may reduce undesirable conduct. Cyproterone acetate, an anti-androgen which also lowers testosterone levels and appears to reduce sexual drive, can be effective. The butyrophenone benperidol has been recommended for the reduction of deviant antisocial sexual behaviour but is not of proven value.

When the unwanted behaviour is not sex-drive dependent, as in the older male, drugs which reduce sex drive are not likely to work. Drugs should be combined with psychological treatment aimed at increasing the patient's motivation to alter behaviour and improve self-control. Aside from anxiety and sexual-drive reduction, drugs have little part to play in treating other disorders of sexuality.

21 Weight changes

Underweight

Loss of weight is a common, non-specific symptom of much serious mental and physical disease, normally one symptom among many. There is, however, one group of conditions collectively labelled 'eating disorders' in which loss of weight is the focus of concern. The most extreme form is anorexia nervosa, in which loss of weight results from self-starvation. The patient refuses to eat, even if hungry, or eats only a little protein food but avoids carbohydrate and fat, secretly vomits after eating, takes purges and diuretics, or exercises to excess in an attempt to lose weight. Such patients have fears of being too fat, or of gaining weight, or of developing a normal sexually mature figure and are determined to stay thin to the point of endangering their lives. They may have a distorted body image, tending to overestimate their size. Anorexics are quite prepared to give false reports of weight gain and lie about themselves to allay concern about their condition. In adolescent girls and young women, anorexia nervosa is accompanied by amenorrhoea and other somatic effects of starvation. But anorexia with refusal to eat an adequate amount of food does also occur, although much less often, in adolescent boys and in older women and men. There is frequently a disturbed relationship with a family member, usually a parent. Refusal to eat may be used to punish another or to attract special concern.

Since extreme weight-loss predisposes to pneumonia, to

gastric dilation, and the patient dying of self-starvation, re-feeding is urgent. It must be carried out away from family pressures, in hospital and without home leave. Nurses who are firm, friendly, and aware of the deceptions such patients may practice can produce weight gain with the help of food supplements alone. Sometimes drugs are necessary to assist psychological treatment. Chlorpromazine (150–300 mg daily) stimulates appetite and causes weight gain. Amitriptyline is occasionally prescribed in the belief that there is an atypical depressive illness to be treated; amitriptyline, like chlorpromazine, has appetite-stimulating and weight-gaining effects over a period.

Bulimia nervosa, with a morbid fear of becoming fat, is characterised by an urge to overeat followed by self-induced vomiting, purging, exercising and other measures to prevent weight gain. It is almost exclusively a disorder of women. More so than anorexia nervosa, bulimia may affect older women and some who are married with children. Treatment is based largely on cognitive–behavioural therapy or various forms of psychotherapy. Drug treatment with antidepressants including the SSRIs may be helpful in combination with cognitive–behavioural therapy, at least in the first few months. Fluoxetine has been used in doses of up to 60 mg daily, and shown to be beneficial even in those who were not depressed. Phenelzine has also been shown to be of benefit.

Pathophysiology

Human appetite involves the transmitters noradrenaline and dopamine, and satiety is thought to involve serotonin (5-HT). There is evidence of abnormal cerebral serotonin function in the eating disorders, with reduced turnover of 5-HT and dopamine, as judged by cerebrospinal fluid levels of their metabolites in bulimia, and abnormal neuroendocrine responses to L-tryptophan in people who lose weight.

Overweight

The psychiatrist encounters overweight as a result of long-term medication with phenothiazines, depot antipsychotics, certain antidepressants and lithium. With these drugs it is thought that blockade of 5-HT receptors is important in producing increased food intake, but dopamine receptor blockade may also contribute to weight gain.

Occasionally, an affective illness results in weight gain instead of loss, and an anxiety state causes 'comfort' overeating. Rarely, refractory obesity, thought to be 'psychological' after defying medical and surgical efforts, is referred to the psychiatrist.

A simple measure of body weight is Body Mass Index (BMI), the weight in kg divided by the square of the height in metres. If over 30, there is Grade II or 'clinically relevant' obesity; over 40 is Grade III or crippling obesity. In a study of patients on long-term antipsychotic medication, 30% had Grade II and 5% had Grade III obesity.

Obesity induced by psychotropic drugs nearly always disappears gradually after the drug is stopped. But stopping the drug may be inadvisable because of the risk of relapse. For lithium, a reduction in the daily dose may be tried, risking relapse for a slimmer figure, or carbamazepine, which does not cause weight gain, substituted. A slimming diet may help, preferably with the advice of a dietician. Often, however, obesity is the price of drug control of positive symptoms of a psychosis, contributing to the characteristic clinical picture of the long-term patient. Obesity resulting from a depressive illness almost always disappears after successful treatment; the SSRIs do not stimulate food intake and for some patients this is an advantage over older drugs.

The treatment of gross obesity with a suspected psychological cause should be approached by investigating for evidence of overeating induced by anxiety, depression or disturbed interpersonal relations. Treatment directed at these conditions, including the appropriate psychotropic drugs, sometimes reduces weight.

The appetite-suppressing drugs, phentermine, diethylpropion and mazindol, which are central stimulants related to amphetamine, are potentially addictive and should not be prescribed. Fenfluramine ('Ponderax'), a serotonin releaser with a sedative action and less addictive, can be prescribed in severe obesity but not for longer than three months. D-Fenfluramine is the active isomer and is available as 'Adifax' (see p. 286). A two-month trial might result in a loss of 8 kg, after which the lost weight is often regained unless the treatment plan includes firmly planned dietary restriction. Treatment should be stopped gradually as sudden discontinuation may cause depression. It must not be combined with an MAOI, because of the risk of the serotonin syndrome (see p. 56). Psychotropic drugs have at present no place in the long-term treatment of chronic obesity. A behavioural approach or a group like 'Weight Watchers', which encourages reducing food intake and increasing energy output over the long-term, can be successful.

Special weighing

It is worth knowing that total starvation will not produce a daily weight loss of more than 500 g in a sedentary person receiving water only; and that excessive feeding will not add more than a maximum of 200 g a day to the body's fat and flesh weight. Larger changes over 24 hours are due to losses or gains of body fluid (losses through urine, sweat or diarrhoea, perhaps). Emptying the bladder of overnight urine, volume 600 ml, means a weight loss of 600 g. Eating dinner will immediately add 500 g to body weight, drinks apart (these are rough values).

Accurate weighing is important in certain clinical conditions and in medical research. The instrument must be reliable and cantilever scales are required. Weighing someone several times a day can be a check on whether an anorexic or bulimic patient has been eating normally or not. In patients prone to excessive water drinking (polydipsia, leading to water intoxication) comparison of the body weight at midday and 4 p.m. with that at 8 a.m. may reveal the extent of overdrinking and the approach to the danger zone of hyponatraemia (below 120 mmol/l). A weight gain of 7% on the early morning body weight is the permitted maximum. In the rare Prader-Willi syndrome (obesity, poor growth, failure of sexual maturation, mental retardation), where the child or adolescent will rob refrigerators and break down doors to get excessive food, frequent weighing can be used to detect the food intake and monitor the effect of treatment.

Further reading

AGRES, W. S., ROSSITER, E. M., ARNOW, B., *et al* (1992) Pharmacologic and cognitive behavioural treatment for bulimia nervosa: a controlled comparison. *American Journal of Psychiatry*, **149**, 82–87.

FLUOXETINE BULIMIA NERVOSA COLLABORATIVE STUDY GROUP (1992) Fluoxetine in the treatment of bulimia nervosa: a multicentre, placebo-controlled, double-blind trial. *Archives of General Psychiatry*, **49**, 139–147.

GOODWIN, G. M., SHAPIRO, C. M., BENNIE, J., *et al* (1989) The neuroendocrine responses and psychological effects of infusion of L-tryptophan in anorexia nervosa. *Psychological Medicine*, **19**, 857–864.

SILVERSTONE, T., SMITH, G. & GOODALL, E. (1988) The prevalence of obesity in patients receiving depot antipsychotics. *British Journal of Psychiatry*, **153**, 214–217.

Part III. Drugs used

22 Antidepressants: monoamine reuptake inhibitors

Amitriptyline and imipramine, introduced in 1957, are two of the oldest and best known drugs for treating depressive illness. Their chemical structure, three joined rings of atoms with a centrally-attached tail or side-chain going off on one side, is termed tricyclic (Fig. 2). The central ring has seven atoms (not six as in phenothiazines), a structure which makes the molecule 'V'-shaped and unable to lie flat. The tricyclic central ring structure makes the drug antidepressant: the side-chain influences potency and sedative action. Tricyclics are not only antidepressants: cyproheptadine ('Periactin') is used as an appetite stimulant; carbamazepine ('Tegretol') as an anticonvulsant, as well as an antimanic and a prophylactic against bipolar affective illness.

The wide range of tricyclics available to choose from is the result of minor structural modifications of the fundamental molecular ground plan. They are called tricyclics because their molecules are made essentially of three linked rings of atoms. If a fourth ring is added, for instance at right angles to the other three, as in maprotiline or mianserin, then the compound is called tetracyclic. Other new antidepressants such as trazodone or the SSRIs have different structures, without tricyclic rings. These drugs have in common the ability to increase the concentration of noradrenaline, 5-HT, or dopamine in the synaptic cleft, and achieve this mainly by blocking the reuptake process (see p. 31). They are therefore known collectively as monoamine reuptake inhibitors (MARIs).

The tricyclics have a number of shortcomings. Their antidepressant effect is slow to develop, taking one to six weeks, they are effective in only a proportion of patients,

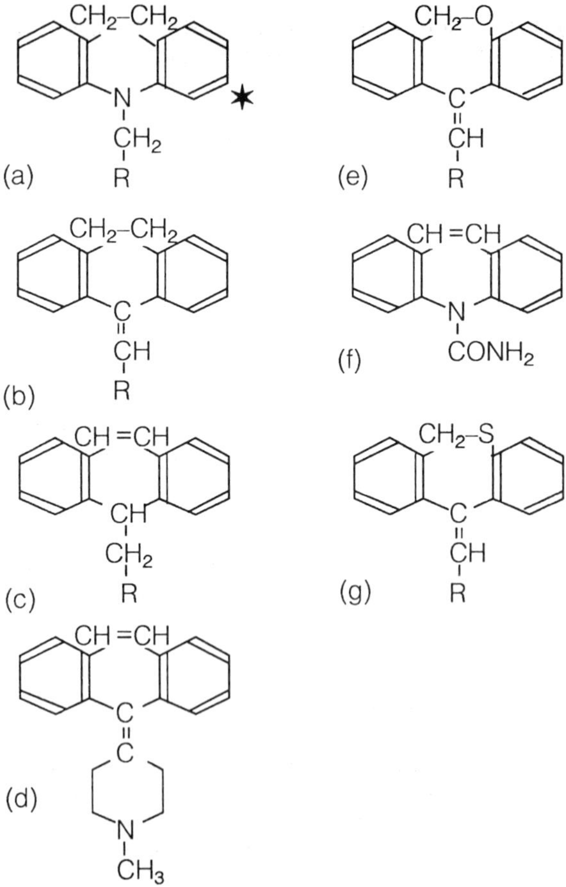

*Fig. 3 Tricyclic drug structures. (a) For imipramine, R is –CH$_2$CH$_2$N(CH$_3$)$_2$; for desipramine, R is –CH$_2$CH$_2$N(CH$_3$)H; for trimipramine, R is –CH(CH$_3$)–CH$_2$N(CH$_3$)$_2$; when a chlorine atom instead of a hydrogen atom is attached to the carbon marked * in the imipramine structure, clomipramine is formed. (b) For amitriptyline, R is as for imipramine; for nortriptyline, R is as for desipramine. (c) For protriptyline, R is as for desipramine. (d) Cyproheptadine, (e) doxepin, (f) carbamazepine, and (g) dothiepin (in e and g R is as imipramine)*

they have many pharmacological side-effects, and are cardiotoxic in overdose. Newer drugs have been developed in the hope of overcoming these problems. Those so far available are less toxic in overdose and have a different pattern of side-effects, which are sometimes better tolerated by patients.

Pharmacological side-effects

Pharmacological side-effects are not necessarily a disadvantage in an antidepressant. For instance, night-time sedation is useful for those patients in whom insomnia is a symptom of their illness, and dryness of the mouth can be a useful biological marker of the adequacy of dose with amitriptyline or imipramine. However, some side-effects are particularly intolerable and may either cause complications or lead the patient to discontinue treatment, with consequent failure to improve, prolongation of illness, and the need for alternative treatment.

In addition to blocking the reuptake of monoamines, these drugs have other pharmacological actions which can be related to particular patterns of side-effects in the following ways.

Anticholinergic effects

Blockade of acetylcholine muscarinic receptors causes a variety of side-effects. Reduced salivation leads to dry mouth and may exacerbate gum disease and dental caries. The pre-existing constipation of the depressed patient is worsened. In high doses or in the elderly, paralytic ileus may occur. Urinary hesitancy occurs, especially in males, and acute retention may develop if the prostate is enlarged.

Blurred vision, with difficulty in accommodating, is a common but not usually severe side-effect. The precipitation of acute narrow angle glaucoma is serious but rare.

Cognitive impairment by this mechanism is not uncommon in the elderly, and confusional states may occur. Those with pre-existing cholinergic deficits due to Alzheimer's disease may be more susceptible to this side-effect.

Tardive dyskinesia tends to be made worse by anti-cholinergic drugs, though not caused by them.

These side-effects are particularly common with amitriptyline, imipramine and clomipramine, less so with dothiepin, lofepramine and maprotiline. The newer drugs – mianserin, trazodone and the serotonin specific reuptake inhibitors (SSRIs), fluvoxamine, fluoxetine, paroxetine and sertraline – do not block muscarinic receptors, but sertraline (or its metabolites) does produce dry mouth.

Histamine H-1 blockade

Histamine H-1 blockade underlies night-time sedation, but also impairs psychomotor coordination during the daytime. It is associated with falls in the elderly and with cognitive slowing. Drugs such as amitriptyline, dothiepin and mianserin are sedatives. Maprotiline, imipramine and nortriptyline are less so. Lofepramine, desipramine and the SSRIs cause little blockade of histamine receptors, but drowsiness is a side-effect of the SSRIs in some patients.

Noradrenaline alpha-1 receptor blockade

Noradrenaline alpha-1 receptor blockade leads to postural hypotension, which may cause dizziness and falls, especially in the elderly; it is also thought to contribute to ejaculatory delay or impotence. This action is strong with amitriptyline, clomipramine, imipramine, mianserin and trazodone. It is weak with dothiepin, maprotiline, nortriptyline and lofepramine and does not occur with viloxazine or the SSRIs. A comparative study of nortriptyline and imipramine in the elderly showed that nortriptyline produced less postural hypotension.

Priapism can occur with trazodone; the mechanism is not certain, though this drug blocks presynaptic alpha-2 receptors, as well as having various other mechanisms. If it occurs the drug should be stopped.

Blockade of serotonin receptors

Serotonin receptors are now classified into at least three main types (see p. 32). 5-HT antagonists, such as cyproheptadine, tend to increase appetite and body weight, and it is probably by this mechanism that antidepressants such as amitriptyline and mianserin cause excessive weight gain, which is lost again when the drug is stopped. This side-effect is not a problem with the SSRIs. Carbohydrate craving can occur as a dose-related side-effect of amitriptyline.

Reuptake inhibition

The older tricyclic antidepressants, imipramine and amitriptyline, block both 5-HT and noradrenaline reuptake; their demethylated metabolites, desipramine and nortriptyline, are more specific as noradrenaline reuptake inhibitors. Clomipramine is the most specific of the older drugs for blockade of the reuptake of 5-HT, as opposed to noradrenaline or dopamine, whereas maprotiline is the most selective noradrenaline reuptake inhibitor. Nomifensine, which is no longer in clinical use, was more specific for blockade of the reuptake of dopamine – a property which is likely to produce activating effects and to risk precipitating psychosis.

Blockade of noradrenaline uptake tends to produce sympathomimetic effects such as tachycardia, and therefore to act synergistically with the anticholinergic effects which block the parasympathetic component of the autonomic nervous system.

Serotonin reuptake inhibition

The development of the SSRIs has provided a clearer picture of the side-effects that are attributable to serotonin reuptake inhibition. The most common side-effects emerging specifically with these drugs have been nausea, diarrhoea, sexual dysfunction, reduced appetite and akathisia.

Although these drugs do not block histamine receptors, drowsiness or somnolence can occur. At higher doses both insomnia and drowsiness occur more commonly. The incidence of nausea, anxiety, anorexia, diarrhoea and tremor also increase with larger doses.

The side-effects of anorgasmia and ejaculatory difficulties were previously noted with clomipramine and occur with the SSRIs. Cyproheptadine taken two hours earlier can counteract this problem. Much more rarely the side-effects of yawning and spontaneous orgasm may occur.

The interactions of SSRIs with the basal ganglia can produce extrapyramidal motor syndromes including akathisia, and may reveal tardive dyskinesia in patients who previously received antipsychotics.

The 'serotonin syndrome' is a serious toxic interaction which is likely to occur when a serotonin reuptake inhibitor is combined with another drug potentiating 5-HT transmission, such as L-tryptophan, lithium or a monoamine oxidase inhibitor. It consists of severe myoclonus with hyperpyrexia, sweating, epileptic seizures and coma (see p. 56). Recovery occurs only in the milder cases but is then complete.

Side-effects with unclear or complex pharmacology

A fine tremor occurs with the tricyclic drugs and to a similar extent with the SSRIs. Propranolol reduces this side-effect but blocks both noradrenaline beta receptors and 5-HT receptors, and the underlying mechanism of the tremor is uncertain.

Excessive sweating occurs to a greater extent with imipramine than with the SSRIs, indicating that the mechanism is complex. Inappropriate secretion of antidiuretic hormone (ADH) has been reported with dothiepin, fluoxetine and lofepramine.

Muscular twitching (myoclonus) occurs with the tricyclic antidepressants and with the newer drugs.

Epileptic fits occur in a dose-dependent manner with the tricyclic antidepressants, up to 1% of patients being affected by higher doses. The mechanism of this effect of antidepressants is not known, but maprotiline is particularly liable to cause it. Drugs with less ictogenic potential include viloxazine and possibly the SSRIs. Existing epilepsy is not necessarily worsened by treatment with MARIs.

The development of mania or rapid cycling bipolar disorder during the course of antidepressant treatment is more likely to occur when there is a previous history of mania. This has been reported with both the tricyclic antidepressants and the newer drugs.

Membrane-stabilising activity

Many centrally-acting drugs have membrane-stabilising or local anaesthetic properties at high doses. This action is responsible for cardiac dysrhythmias associated with overdoses of antidepressants, and can lead to asystole and fatal outcome in suicide attempts. This mechanism of action is unrelated to either the anticholinergic effects or any of the other properties discussed above. Thus, in spite of its low anticholinergic properties, a drug such as dothiepin owes its lethality in overdose to this membrane-stabilising property. Antidepressants with weaker membrane-stabilising activity include mianserin, viloxazine, lofepramine, and the four SSRIs. These drugs should be used if an antidepressant is required in a patient with cardiac disease, especially one with a conduction defect or after a myocardial infarction. However, the occurrence of ectopic beats is not a contraindication to use of the tricyclic drugs; the membrane-stabilising activity may in fact reduce the number of ectopics in such patients.

Drop-outs from treatment

Most side-effects are dose- and age-related and some, for instance nausea with the SSRIs, tend to decrease with continued treatment. Thus the risk of drop-outs may be reduced by starting on a lower dose, especially in the elderly. In research studies of the newer drugs, a smaller proportion of patients discontinued treatment because of side-effects compared with the older tricyclic antidepressants, imipramine or amitriptyline. Thus about 20% discontinued tricyclic treatment compared with 15% with the SSRIs: 5% of patients on placebo dropped out because of new symptoms. Among the tricyclic drugs, lofepramine produces fewer side-effects and is much less cardiotoxic.

Toxic and allergic side-effects

These are generally rare and only detected after the drug had been marketed and several thousand patients treated. Patients on mianserin should have monthly blood tests for the first three months; the risk of bone marrow disorder is about 1 in 5000, and the elderly are particularly at risk.

Because of the risk of fatal systemic vasculitis, fluoxetine should be stopped if a rash develops. Abnormal liver function tests occur occasionally with many antidepressants; most are unpredictable and independent of dose, and their potential severity varies widely. Previous exposure to enzyme-inducing agents may increase the rate of formation of reactive drug metabolites, and potentiate hepatotoxicity. Anticonvulsants and chronic alcohol ingestion may be important in this respect. With lofepramine, jaundice may develop in the first eight weeks but is reversible on discontinuing the drug.

Overdoses

Overdoses of most tricyclics lead, in one to five hours, to unconsciousness, with a catastrophic fall in blood pressure, cardiac arrhythmias, epileptic fits, and sometimes status epilepticus. Stomach washout, control of fits, maintenance of blood pressure and hence of kidney function must be carried out in a medical ward under specialist advice. Prognosis is good where treatment begins shortly after the overdose. The SSRIs are relatively safe in overdose but can cause vomiting, agitation and fits.

Drug interactions

The tricyclics interfere with the control of blood pressure by adrenergic blocking drugs, such as guanethidine, which have to be taken up into nerve endings in order to act. They also potentiate the action of adrenaline in local anaesthetics by preventing adrenaline reuptake, thereby causing a rise in blood pressure. Substances which activate the liver mono-oxygenase enzyme system, carbamazepine, barbiturates, phenytoin and nicotine, may lower the plasma concentration of tricyclic antidepressants. Oestrogens inhibit the metabolism of tricyclic antidepressants leading to higher plasma levels. Cimetidine also raises the plasma concentration of tricyclics. Many antipsychotic drugs increase the plasma concentration of tricyclics by inhibiting the hydroxylase enzymes in the liver. The SSRIs to varying extents also inhibit the hydroxylase enzymes.

Withdrawal reactions

Withdrawal reactions after tricyclic antidepressants include nausea, vomiting, sweating and insomnia lasting for a few days.

With the SSRIs withdrawal problems are uncommon but paroxetine has been associated with dizziness, sweating and tremor.

Clinical effectiveness

The tricyclics at doses of 125–150 mg daily or above are effective in the treatment of depressive illness, especially moderate or severe cases. Amitriptyline and imipramine have been studied most extensively, other tricyclics less so. The newer drugs have generally to be shown to be superior to placebo before they are marketed. Many but not all have been shown to be of equal efficacy to the older drugs. The choice of drugs should therefore be based upon the pattern of symptoms and the likely tolerability of side-effects for the individual patient.

Mechanism of antidepressant effect

The MARIs act primarily by blocking the reuptake of noradrenaline, 5-HT and to some extent dopamine, thus increasing the concentration of these transmitters in the synaptic cleft. Some, such as mianserin and trazodone, achieve this also by blocking pre-synaptic noradrenaline alpha-2 auto-receptors, thereby increasing the release of noradrenaline. Their other actions, blocking receptors for acetylcholine, histamine, noradrenaline and serotonin, are thought to account for side-effects but not for clinical efficacy.

The long delay in the antidepressant effect suggests that adaptive processes are important in the mechanism of action. It is known that changes occur in the transmitter receptors. Thus noradrenaline beta and alpha-2 receptors are gradually reduced in number (down-regulated) during antidepressant treatment. Slow changes occur too in both pre- and post-synaptic serotonin receptors and alpha-1 receptors which are up-regulated. Other slow processes which may be set in train include the transport of enzymes from the cell body of the neurone along the axon to the nerve endings. These enzymes are involved in the synthesis of transmitters and the neuropeptide modulators. Although the basis of the antidepressant effect is not understood, the available evidence suggests that the overall effect of antidepressants is to increase transmission at noradrenaline and 5-HT synapses. If the patient who has recovered on antidepressant treatment is given a diet which is deficient in the amino acid tryptophan, and designed to deplete brain 5-HT, they experience a resurgence of depressive symptoms.

Tricyclic antidepressants

Amitriptyline is described in detail as the typical tricyclic drug. This does not mean we regard it as pre-eminent, we could equally well have placed imipramine in this position. To avoid tiresome repetition of shared properties, other tricyclics are only briefly described.

The most common cause of failure to relieve depressive illness with a drug is to use too small a dose. As long as side-effects are small, the dose can be raised. A second cause is impatience: at least two weeks' action is needed and the patient must be aware of this.

Amitriptyline

Amitriptyline ('Tryptizol', 'Lentizol') may be used for:

  (a) depressive illness especially with 'biological symptoms'
  (b) for anxiety states
  (c) for nocturnal enuresis in children.

For adults, start with oral tablets after food, 10 mg or 25 mg thrice daily, or simply 50–100 mg at night since then a separate hypnotic may not be needed, and morning anxiety and agitation will be better controlled. After two days the dose can be raised, and raised again as required. A daily dose of 150 mg is quite usual. There will be no response for at least two weeks, and some patients will need to go to 300 mg daily to improve. Individuals differ in their tolerance of side-effects but it usually increases in a few days, which is the reason for starting with low doses and raising by steps. If side-effects continue to be a problem, try a different tricyclic. Where agitation and insomnia remain poorly controlled, small doses of a phenothiazine such as chlorpromazine, or a benzodiazepine such as temazepam or diazepam, may be a helpful addition.

Adults who say they get indigestion or vomiting with tablets may try syrup instead. Slow-release preparations probably have no advantage over tablets in similar dose and may be more expensive.

Antidepressants must be continued for some time after recovery. For how long is uncertain, but, in general, advise the patient to continue treatment for six months after they are better. Then reduce the dose in steps. If depressive symptoms begin to return, go back to the original higher dose and try reduction again in another three months. Do not be in a hurry to stop treatment. After a third attack in three years, prophylaxis by continuing the tricyclic is a reasonable line of treatment, but the drug may need to be continued at the dose level found therapeutic and not reduced. Alternatively, lithium may be given (see p. 229). The decision when to start prophylaxis, and when to stop it, depends on weighing the social consequences of a further depression, its likely severity, the risk of suicide, the side-effects of the drug and the patient's motivation.

A similar approach is used for panic attacks and phobias. In these it is important to start with very low doses, as there may be an initial worsening. The dose should be gradually increased to similar levels as for depression. In children, amitriptyline reduces frequency of bed-wetting: 25 or 50 mg at night. It is less effective and more upsetting than an electric alarm and should not be used where incontinence has physical illness as its cause (see Chapter 15 – Disorders of childhood).

Brain damage in children and in adults is no contraindication to tricyclic treatment, and depression after a stroke can respond well to the drug. Heart damage, however, in particular myocardial infarction, carries some risk of dysrhythmia with a tricyclic, and a different drug or electroconvulsive therapy at 12 weeks or more from the attack may be safer. Tricyclics, in therapeutic dose, are not toxic to the healthy heart, but stabilised treatment for hypertension may be upset.

Side-effects

These are quick (within hours) or slow (after two weeks or more of treatment). The quick are very common: drowsiness, over-sedation, indigestion, dry mouth, constipation, blurring of vision, headache, dizziness and postural hypotension, and difficulty in urination. The slow, in order of increasing rarity, are weight gain (lost again when drug is stopped), shaking of limbs (myoclonus), hypomania, grand mal attack, toxic hallucinosis (like that from anticholinergics), paralytic ileus causing acute abdominal pain, Parkinsonian tremor with facial immobility and stiff movements. The last is more likely when lithium also is taken.

Patients on monoamine oxidase inhibitor (MAOI) drugs or who have taken them in the previous seven days run the risk, when given amitriptyline (or other amine tricyclics), of developing a severe vascular headache with high blood pressure. Treat with phentolamine (5–10 mg intravenously). But combined MAOI-tricyclic therapy for resistant depression is possible (see p. 78).

Note that some phenothiazine drugs, given concurrently with a tricyclic, inhibit its metabolism and raises its blood level in consequence.

Preparations

Tablets: 10, 25, 50 mg
Capsules: 75 mg
Sustained release capsules ('Lentizol'): 25, 50 mg
Syrup: 10 mg/5 ml
Injection: ampoule of 10 ml contains 10 mg/ml

Nortriptyline

The clinical effects are like those of amitriptyline, except that nortriptyline ('Allegron', 'Aventyl') has little sedative or hypnotic action and produces less postural hypotension. In fact, amitriptyline is rapidly metabolised in the body to nortriptyline so it is not surprising if the two are similar. Doses can, however, be a little lower – 75 mg daily may be enough, producing a plasma concentration of 50–150 ng/ml or about 200–600 mmol/l.

Preparations

Tablets: 10, 25 mg
Capsules: 10, 25 mg
Liquid: 10 mg/5 ml

Imipramine, desipramine, trimipramine

Very like amitriptyline but less sedative, imipramine ('Tofranil') can be used in the same way in the same doses, up to 300 mg daily. Desipramine is the metabolite of imipramine, but is less sedative still; it is rather expensive. Trimipramine differs by one carbon atom in the side-chain from imipramine; it is more sedative but otherwise has very similar properties. Desipramine is the most specific of this group for blocking noradrenaline as opposed to 5-HT reuptake.

Preparations

Imipramine –
   tablets: 10, 25 mg
   syrup: 25 mg/5 ml
   injection: ampoule of 2 ml contains 25 mg
Desipramine –
   tablets: 25 mg ('Pertofran') (up to 200 mg daily)
Trimipramine –
   tablets:10, 25 mg ('Surmontil') (up to 300 mg daily)
   capsules: 50 mg

Dothiepin

Dothiepin ('Prothiaden') resembles amitriptyline in its sedative and antidepressant effect, but is less potent, so that a minimum of 100 mg daily must be given to have more than a placebo effect. It has fewer autonomic side-effects and is therefore more suitable for the elderly. However, in overdose it is at least as cardiotoxic as amitriptyline.

Preparations

Tablets: 75 mg
Capsules: 25 mg

Clomipramine

Clomipramine ('Anafranil') is imipramine with one chlorine atom added to a side ring. It is the most specific of the tricyclic drugs for blocking 5-HT rather than noradrenaline reuptake. It is also anticholinergic, sedative and produces postural hypotension. It is slightly more potent than imipramine and the doses should be correspondingly lower, being built up to 30–150 mg daily. It is used for depressive illnesses in general, but has also been recommended for depressions resistant to ordinary treatments, when combined with lithium carbonate to produce a plasma level of 0.5–0.8 mmol/l. Formerly, L-tryptophan was included in the combination but this was withdrawn because of eosinophiliamyalgia. Clomipramine must not be combined with or used within three weeks of MAOIs (see p. 78).

It is available by intramuscular injection and also by intravenous infusion, the only tricyclic drug suitable for this method. Intravenous infusion should be given only to patients who are unable to take the drug orally.

Clomipramine has also been used with good effect with obsessional and phobic illness, even without accompanying depression. The dose is generally higher than that used in depression, being built up to 100–150 mg daily over the course of two weeks. Many patients with panic disorders tend to experience intensified anxiety during the first few days of treatment, and therefore the dosage of clomipramine should be built up gradually.

Clomipramine may, particularly at night, provoke a drug-induced delirious psychosis, which disappears within a few days of stopping the drug.

Clomipramine is not very suitable for patients with liver damage or cardiac conditions. With the development of the SSRIs, clomipramine can be replaced by the latter for most patients.

Preparations

Capsules: 10, 25, 50 mg
Sustained release tablet: 75 mg
Syrup: 25 mg/5 ml
Injection: 2 ml ampoule contains 25 mg

Mianserin and trazodone

Mianserin ('Bolvidon', 'Norval') and trazodone ('Molipaxin') are 5-HT reuptake inhibitors but also block noradrenaline alpha-2 receptors, 5-HT and histamine receptors. They are sedative and produce weight gain. Their advantages are the lack of anticholinergic side-effects and their relative lack of cardiotoxicity. They interfere with the actions of clonidine but are not known to interfere with the actions of other anti-hypertensive drugs. Trazodone is commenced in a dose of 150 mg, increasing to 300 mg, taken at night. There have been rare reports of it producing priapism, and it should be stopped if persistent erections occur spontaneously.

Mianserin is commenced with 30 mg, increasing up to 90 mg, taken at night. Bone marrow depression with agranulocytosis occurs in about 1 in 5000 patients. This is more common in the elderly, tending to occur after four to six weeks of treatment, and is usually reversible.

A full blood count is recommended every four weeks during the first three months of treatment. Subsequently, if the patient develops fever, sore throat or stomatitis the blood count should be repeated and the treatment stopped. Arthralgia, polyarthropathy and rashes may also occur.

Preparations

Mianserin –
    tablets: 10, 20, 30 mg
Trazodone –
    tablets: 50, 100, 150 mg
    liquid for oral use: 50 mg/ml

Lofepramine

Lofepramine ('Gamanil') is a tricyclic antidepressant that is non-sedative and has less anticholinergic side-effects and less cardiotoxicity than other tricyclics. It is metabolised to desipramine. It can produce hypotension and tachycardia.

Jaundice may develop in the first eight weeks but is reversible on discontinuing the drug.

Among the tricyclics this appears to be the safest in overdose. The usual dose starts with 70 mg, increasing to 210 mg daily, depending upon response.

Preparations

Tablets: 70 mg

Serotonin-specific reuptake inhibitors

Four drugs are currently available which are relatively specific in blocking 5-HT reuptake, having few other pharmacological actions. These are fluvoxamine ('Faverin'), fluoxetine ('Prozac'), paroxetine ('Seroxat') and sertraline ('Lustral').

These drugs have been shown to be effective in depressive illness and in the prevention of recurrences of depression. They are also thought to be effective in anxiety states, including panic disorder where fluvoxamine is superior to specific noradrenaline reuptake inhibitors, and in bulimia nervosa, where fluoxetine has been found to reduce bulimic episodes.

They share the same profile of side-effects, with few differences. However, sertraline produces more dry mouth, and paroxetine seems more liable to cause drowsiness.

Their main side-effects are nausea, diarrhoea, somnolence, insomnia, anxiety or agitation, tremor and sexual dysfunction. Extrapyramidal symptoms including akathisia and dystonia can occur and there is a risk of fits occurring.

Rashes occurring with fluoxetine should lead to discontinuation of the drug because of the risk of severe vasculitis. Dyspnoea with fluoxetine may indicate the development of a rare pulmonary inflammation.

Suicidal preoccupations and violent behaviour may occur as an idiosyncratic reaction in a small number of patients, although in general the drugs reduce suicidal behaviour.

The drugs should be used cautiously in patients with liver or renal disease, and avoided in pregnancy and breast feeding. Their use in children has not been elucidated.

They may be useful in combination with lithium, but should then be monitored for side-effects, including lithium toxicity and serotonin syndrome; convulsions and raised temperature should lead to cessation of treatment.

The drugs should not be combined with MAOIs. An interval of two weeks should elapse between the use of fluvoxamine, paroxetine or sertraline and an MAOI; with fluoxetine there should be an interval of five weeks before an MAOI is commenced. Likewise, the drugs should not be given until at least two weeks have elapsed after an MAOI has been stopped.

The control of diabetes may be altered by fluoxetine.

The drugs appear to differ mainly in their pharmacokinetics. Thus fluoxetine has the longest elimination half-life (two to three days) and is metabolised to norfluoxetine which is similarly active and has a half-life of seven to nine days. This is a disadvantage if side-effects develop, or there is an interaction with other drugs such as MAOIs.

The elimination half-lives of fluvoxamine, paroxetine and sertraline range from 15–30 hours. Thus a steady-state plasma level is reached after about five to seven days with them, but after one to two months with fluoxetine.

The drugs tend to inhibit liver hydroxylase enzymes leading to higher levels of tricyclic antidepressants, phenothiazines, and certain anti-arrhythmics. Sertraline may be less active in this regard.

Fluvoxamine inhibits oxidase enzymes in the liver and can thereby lead to increases in plasma levels of drugs metabolised by the enzymes. Increased levels of propranolol and warfarin occur. There may also be interactions with phenytoin and theophylline. The other SSRIs have not been fully assessed in this regard and should therefore be used cautiously in combination with the other drugs. No interactions have been seen between fluvoxamine and digoxin or atenolol. Sertraline is 98% bound to plasma proteins and there may be interactions with other drugs that are highly protein bound.

Dosages

Fluoxetine is given in a dose of 20 mg daily for depression. A dose of up to 60 mg daily is recommended for bulimia nervosa.

Fluvoxamine is commenced in a dose of 50–100 mg in the evening, increasing to 150–300 mg daily in divided doses.

Sertraline is commenced in a dose of 50 mg daily with food, and increased to 100–150 mg daily.

Paroxetine is commenced in a dose of 20 mg daily in the morning with food. This can be increased by 10 mg increments to a maximum of 50 mg daily.

When the drugs are used for anxiety states, the starting dose should be low because there may be an initial increase in agitation in the first few days.

Preparations

Fluoxetine –
   capsules: 20 mg
Fluvoxamine –
   tablets: 50, 100 mg
Sertraline –
   tablets: 50, 100 mg
Paroxetine –
   tablets: 20, 30 mg

Related drugs

The maximum daily dose is given in brackets in each case.

Protriptyline ('Concordin'), tablets: 5, 10 mg (60 mg)
Butriptyline ('Evadyne'), tablets: 25, 50 mg (150 mg)
Doxepin ('Sinequan'), capsules: 10, 25, 50, 75 mg (300 mg)
Maprotiline ('Ludiomil'), tablets: 10, 25, 50, 75 mg (150 mg)
Iprindole ('Prondol'), tablets: 15, 30 mg (180 mg)
Viloxazine ('Vivalan'), tablets: 50, 150 mg (400 mg)
Amoxapine ('Asendis'), tablets: 25, 50, 100, 150 mg (300 mg)

Drug combinations

These are given for information only: we do not recommend them.

'Limbitrol-10': 25 mg amitriptyline with 10 mg of the
    benzodiazepine 'Librium' (Limbitrol-5 is half-strength)
'Motival': 10 mg nortriptyline with 0.5 mg fluphenazine
    ('Motipress' is similar but three-times stronger)
'Triptafen DA': 25 mg amitriptyline with 2 mg perphenazine
    ('Triptafen-forte' has twice as much perphenazine;
    'Triptafen-minor' has 10 mg amitriptyline with 2 mg
    perphenazine)

23 Antidepressants: monoamine oxidase inhibitors

The discovery of the psychotropic effects of monoamine oxidase inhibitors (MAOIs) dates from 1952 when iproniazid given to patients for tuberculosis was found to lift their mood. Isoniazid, still widely used for patients with tuberculosis, is much less potent as an MAOI, and although it produces psychotic reactions in some patients with tuberculosis, it is thought to do so by a different mechanism. Iproniazid was not introduced as an antidepressant until 1957.

The uses of MAOIs in psychiatry do not fall into neat categories. They have been described as sedatives, euphoriants, antidepressants, and antiphobics. It is more rational, however, to think of them simply as having some slow central nervous modifying action, changing the balance of brain functions in some as yet unknown way: some patients are undoubtedly helped by MAOIs, some even specifically by only one particular drug of the group. The indications are depressive illnesses, especially atypical depressions, anxiety states and where monoamine reuptake inhibitor antidepressants have failed (see p. 78). They are also used in Parkinson's disease.

Most MAOIs are hydrazine derivatives and contain the chemical grouping –NH–NH– in the side-chain. Hydrazines such as phenelzine ('Nardil') are inactivated by acetylation in the liver, by which –NH–NH– is converted to –NH–NH–CO–CH$_3$. Speed of acetylation is genetically determined, some individuals being fast and others slow acetylators.

The non-hydrazine derivatives include amphetamine and more particularly its relative tranylcypromine ('Parnate').

They may be classified by clinical usage in this section of the pharmacopoeia, although by chemistry and metabolism they are distinct.

Most MAOI drugs combine irreversibly with, and thus inactivate the enzymes which oxidise serotonin, noradrenaline, dopamine, tyramine and other amines. These amines may be neurotransmitters, potential toxins in foods, or ingredients of medicines. The enzymes inactivated are found in many parts of the body, for instance the intestinal wall, liver, the platelets of the blood, the heart, kidney and lung, and the brain. The enzymes in different tissues differ in the relative efficiency with which they oxidise different amines, and their relative sensitivities to different MAOI drugs also differ. There are two main enzymes, MAO-A and -B. MAO-A oxidises serotonin and noradrenaline. Both enzymes oxidise dopamine and tyramine. MAO-A is inhibited by moclobemide ('Manerix'), MAO-B by selegiline ('El-depryl'), and both are inhibited by the older MAOIs – phenelzine isocarboxazid and tranylcypromine.

Apart from amine oxidases, the MAOIs inactivate other enzymes, particularly liver hydroxylases. The drugs may also inactivate pyridoxal, a co-enzyme derived from vitamin B6 (pyridoxine), which plays a part in many processes in the metabolism of organic acids and of the neurotransmitter GABA. These inactivations are rapid whereas the clinical effects are slow, so it is difficult to know how the drugs act, and whether their inhibition of monoamine oxidases, simply one among several inhibitions, is what matters.

Within the brain, monoamine oxidase is present pre-synaptically in mitochondria, and in the synaptic cleft where noradrenaline, 5-HT or dopamine are transmitters. It is thought that MAOIs increase the storage and release of these transmitters, and slow their breakdown after release.

Enzymes are proteins which are continually being broken down and resynthesised during life. When an enzyme is irreversibly inhibited and hence functionally destroyed, fresh enzyme gradually resynthesised in the course of two or three weeks eventually replaces all that has been destroyed, unless fresh inhibitor is continually added. In treatment, free MAOI disappears by metabolism and excretion, leaving inactivated enzymes which take time to be replaced. This time for recovery is why it is advisable to wait two weeks after stopping an MAOI before starting another drug (e.g. a tricyclic), and also why measurement of an MAOI drug blood-level may tell little about the degree of enzyme inhibition. The activity of the enzyme in platelets can, however, be usefully measured. The reversible inhibitors of MAO-A (RIMAs), such as moclobemide, allow for a much shorter washout period of only 24 hours.

Because of the protean effects of MAOI, caution and watchfulness are required: caution in deciding to use them and to mix them with other drugs, and watchfulness for the physical signs of side-effects and of toxicity. They are frequently hypotensive, especially in causing postural hypotension, but paradoxically facilitate hypertensive episodes, sometimes with severe headache, particularly when amine-rich foods are eaten. This occurs because amines such as tyramine in food are normally metabolised by monoamine oxidases in the gut wall and liver, and do not reach the general circulation. If they do, they enter sympathetic nerve endings and cause the release of noradrenaline, leading to vasoconstriction, cardiac stimulation and hypertension. The latter can be so severe as to produce cerebral or subarachnoid haemorrhages. Patients should be advised not to eat any cheese, hung-game or caviar, and to avoid pickled herrings, and meat extracts, 'Bovril', 'Oxo', 'Marmite'; alcohol is best avoided, especially heavy red wines but also non-alcoholic beers may cause problems. Bananas, except perhaps the skins, and broad beans, except the pods, are safe.

The MAOIs may cause ankle oedema and puffy hands because of fluid retention. They may be hypoglycaemic because they inhibit the decay of natural insulin. They have caused jaundice. They are unsafe combined with amphetamines, methyldopa and the serotonin agonist buspirone. They prevent the metabolism and so enhance the effect of morphine, pethidine, nefopam and dextromethorphan, and likewise of anti-Parkinsonian drugs, tricyclic antidepressants, barbiturates, and phenytoin. If an MAOI is added to the prescription of a patient already stabilised on one or more of these other drugs, the stability may be upset, and a toxic overdose develop. But the fact remains that, in spite of many potential risks, troubles are uncommon in practice when care is taken.

Patients should carry a card explaining they are taking an MAOI, so that other practitioners, including anaesthetists and dentists, may know and prescribe their drugs with appropriate caution to avoid unpleasant or dangerous interactions.

The selective MAO-A or -B inhibitors produce much less interaction with foodstuffs and other drugs because some compounds including tyramine can be metabolised by either enzyme and, in the case of the RIMAs, because their reversibility means they can be displaced from the enzyme by high levels of substrates such as tyramine.

Phenelzine

Phenelzine ('Nardil') and the related drug isocarboxazid ('Marplan') may be used for:

(a)   depressive states, especially those with atypical features (see p. 78)
(b)   depressions unresponsive to tricyclic drugs, including combined treatment
(c)   anxiety states.

Phenelzine is started with 15 mg thrice daily, and after one week increased to 60 mg daily if side-effects are not marked. Raise to 75 mg daily after a second week, and so continue for at least two weeks. It is possible to give 90 mg daily. Isocarboxazid is commenced at 10 mg, increasing to 30 mg daily. Elderly patients will require lower doses than these. Antidepressant response is slow, taking two to six weeks.

Combination with tricyclics

Depressive illness which has not responded to a tricyclic antidepressant, or MAOI alone, may do so with combined treatment, but only certain tricyclics are safe to combine: either amitriptyline or imipramine may be used. Start the tricyclic antidepressant drug first in a low dose, for example 100 mg at night, or not more than 150 mg daily. Clomipramine or SSRI must not be used. Then introduce phenelzine twice and then thrice daily in usual dose. Inquire carefully for side-effects and measure blood level effects after two or three days, at one, two and three weeks, and whenever the patient is seen thereafter. If the patient is already taking phenelzine it is possible to start a tricyclic with it by small doses at night, increasing very slowly.

Combination with lithium

Drug-resistant depression may respond to phenelzine (15 mg thrice daily), plus lithium carbonate to give plasma lithium 0.5–0.8 mmol/l.

Side-effects and interactions

The drug has some sedative action and may quickly counteract insomnia in some states of tension. It should not be given during infective hepatitis, obstructive jaundice, liver cirrhosis or congestive cardiac failure. It should not be used in cerebrovascular disease and should be used cautiously in the elderly. Patients must be told to avoid all self-medication, for instance for colds, because of the risk of interactions with ephedrine. They should avoid meat or yeast extracts, pickled herrings, chicken liver, some red wines and cheeses, especially highly fermented ones such as Gorgonzola.

Common side-effects are sweating, dry mouth, weakness, and faintness, especially from postural hypotension. Less frequent are tingling paraesthesia in upper or lower limbs (for which pyridoxine, 50 mg daily, is sometimes given), ankle oedema and tremor. Toxic reactions include hyperpyrexia, convulsions, agitation and confusional states in which hallucinations may be prominent. Depressed patients may swing into hypomania while on the drug.

In cases of hypertensive crisis give phentolamine (5–10 mg intravenously).

Because of drug interactions, avoid sympathomimetic amines (amphetamine, fenfluramine, ephedrine), including those sometimes present in proprietary cold cures and cough medicines, antihypertensive drugs (such as methyldopa, guanethidine), and antihistamines. Note that preparations of local anaesthetic sometimes contain sympathomimetic amines.

Sensitivity to insulin may be increased, perhaps by blocking insulin destruction, and hence increasing sensitivity to oral anti-diabetic drugs resulting in unexpected hypoglycaemia. Morphine, pethidine and dextromethorphan (in 'Actifed' cough linctus) are contraindicated, but not other analgesics. The mechanism of the interaction with pethidine is not fully understood, but a 'serotonin syndrome' has been described. Metabolism of many drugs by the liver, for instance barbiturates and phenytoin, may also be interfered with.

Preparations

Phenelzine –
    tablets: 15 mg
Isocarboxazid –
    tablets: 10 mg

Tranylcypromine

Although tranylcypromine ('Parnate') has less marked MAOI activity than phenelzine, it is strongly sympatho-mimetic and has side-effects and interactions similar to phenelzine. The same drugs and foods must be avoided, as hypertensive and other side-effects are not infrequent, but liver damage is less likely.

In a dose of 10 mg twice or thrice daily it is used against depressions where phenelzine might be prescribed. However, like amphetamine, to which it is chemically related, tranylcypromine has some immediate euphoriant effect and may cause insomnia, so is best taken in the morning. The immediate effect encourages the patient, but can lead to dependence.

Preparations

Tablets: 10 mg

Note

A combination of tranylcypromine (10 mg) and the phenothiazine drug trifluoperazine ('Stelazine') (1 mg) under the name 'Parstelin' is sold and is used when sedation is required in addition to antidepressant activity. The evidence for the special value of 'Parstelin' is limited: part of it is by analogy with amphetamine, the effects of which are helpfully modified by combination with amylobarbitone.

Moclobemide

Moclobemide ('Manerix') is a benzamide derivative and a reversible inhibitor of monoamine oxidase-A (RIMA). Tyramine taken with it can still be metabolised by MAO-B. Also because of its reversibility, large quantities of tyramine or other substrates will displace moclobemide from the enzyme. It is thus relatively free of interactions with foodstuffs but patients should avoid large quantities of tyramine-rich foods and certain drugs (see below).

Moclobemide is an effective antidepressant in doses of 300 mg daily or more. Its use in anxiety states is currently being investigated.

Side-effects are less common than with the older MARIs and include insomnia, headache, dizziness and nausea. It may cause reversible confusional states. It is not sedative, lacks anticholinergic effects, and is relatively safe in overdose. Because of its reversibility and short half-life, a switch to other drugs can be made after only 24 hours. However, it should not be started after an MARI which blocks serotonin reuptake until the other drug has had time to leave the body (four to five half-lives).

Start on 300 mg daily with food, adjusting the dose to 150–600 mg daily according to response. The drug is metabolised in the liver and lower doses are not required in patients with renal disease or the physically well elderly. In hepatic disease, lower doses are needed.

Interactions

It is metabolised by hepatic mono-oxygenase, and blood levels are increased by drugs such as cimetidine, so that a lower dose is needed. Patients should avoid cough remedies containing drugs like ephedrine, or dextromethorphan. Pethidine and codeine should not be administered with it, and other opiates should be used with caution. Of the MARIs, clomipramine and the SSRIs must be avoided (see p. 206).

Preparation

Tablets: 150 mg

Selegiline

Selegiline ('Eldepryl') is a selective MAO-B inhibitor which potentiates dopamine function in the brain. It is used in Parkinson's disease, but has not been found useful as an antidepressant. It does not produce the tyramine reaction and no diet restrictions are required.

The side-effects include hypotension and nausea and it can cause confusional states and psychotic reactions, as might be expected from its potentiation of dopamine transmission.

Particular interest surrounds selegiline because of the occurrence of a Parkinson-like condition caused by the 'synthetic heroin' contaminant MPTP (methyl phenyltetrahydropyridine). MPTP is converted by MAO-B to another compound, MPP, which enters nigrostriatal dopamine neurones selectively, and destroys them. Selegiline gives full protection against this toxic action of MPTP in animals. It has also been found to delay the development of disability in Parkinson's disease.

Preparation

Tablets: 5, 10 mg

Further reading

CALLINGHAM, B. A. (1993) Drug interactions with reversible monoamine oxidase -A inhibitors. *Clinical Neuropharmacology*, **16** (suppl. 2), S42–S50.

24   Lithium

Principally used to treat affective disorders and especially to prevent their recurrence, lithium salts also sometimes suppress schizophrenic symptoms and some states of aggression of uncertain diagnosis, including those in the mentally handicapped; they may also aid in preventing relapse of alcoholism, but this requires further study.

Lithium is widely used in psychiatry and considerable knowledge of its physiology has been obtained. As this has a direct bearing on its clinical use, an extensive account is given here.

Lithium is an element closely related to sodium and potassium (group 1 of the Periodic Table of elements) and like them is found widely distributed as salts in nature, in rocks, spa waters, and in the fluids of plants and animals. Traces are normal in the human body (about one-thousandth of the therapeutic level), and the lithium ion is distributed fairly evenly throughout the body water, intracellular and extracellular. Sodium in contrast is mostly extra- and potassium intra-cellular.

Lithium has an immense number of actions in plants and animals, modifying the development of some, of endocrine functions in others, and of enzyme activities in a wide range of systems, but these activities all depend on particular concentrations of lithium ions. At the dilution present in normal untreated man, or resulting from drinking spa water, lithium can have no clinical effect. Many of the biochemical and biological actions of lithium described from the laboratory on isolated enzymes or organisms in experiments require lithium in many times the concentration achieved in therapy, way beyond the toxic limit in man. Therapeutic, human biochemical changes, and then toxic effects appear in a rather narrow range of concentrations, so that the safe successful use of lithium in psychiatry depends on close control of the amount of lithium circulating in the blood. Understanding how this can vary is essential.

The lithium ion diffuses rapidly, so that it is absorbed from the stomach into the blood and enters most tissues; it soon begins to appear in the urine. It also appears in sweat but not, unless there is diarrhoea or failure of the lithium tablet to disintegrate, in the faeces. Lithium is not significantly stored anywhere in the body and, therefore, the amount circulating in the blood at any time depends only on the balance between the rate of intake by mouth and of excretion in the urine. There is usually both a rapid rate of absorption and a rapid excretion, provided renal function is normal. Lithium is excreted by glomerular filtration, with some reabsorption from the proximal tubule – as for sodium but much less efficiently. Renal blood flow, as decided by blood pressure, degree of vasoconstriction, hydration, and sodium intake, is therefore important. A diet low in sodium, heavy sweating as in hot weather or pyrexia, and hypotension from any cause, decrease urinary lithium and raise it in the blood, on constant oral dosing.

When a tablet of lithium citrate or carbonate is swallowed, providing it disintegrates and dissolves, the lithium concentration in the blood plasma rises rapidly to a sharp peak in 1–4 hours and then falls again, at first steeply and then more gently in an exponential curve, as the lithium diffuses into the tissues or is lost in the urine. The plasma half-life depends on renal excretion and varies from 7–20 hours in physically healthy individuals but is longer in the elderly or physically unwell. On a regular dose, steady-state levels would be reached after between two and nine days. If lithium is taken thrice daily at, say, 8 a.m., 1 p.m. and 6 p.m., the second dose builds on top of the first, and the third on that to produce a very high peak before the fall, which will then last 14 hours. So the blood concentration is swinging between a very high level for a short time, and much lower levels for a considerable time, and is always changing. This has two important practical consequences:

(a) Unpleasant side-effects such as vomiting and diarrhoea, or polydipsia, are produced more by higher levels. Therefore, keep the peaks down.

(b) It is essential to note the time when a blood sample for lithium measurement is taken, and the time when the last dose was taken also. Otherwise, the lithium value obtained by the laboratory cannot be correctly interpreted. To guide treatment the lithium is measured only when it is rather slowly changing near the latter part of its fall. So the blood should be taken at least 8 hours, preferably 12 hours, after the last dose, or just before taking the first dose of the day, if this is more convenient. This gives the minimum concentration of plasma lithium which is being reached on that dose schedule, and treatment is guided by these minima, and not by the heights which may be reached from time to time. On the other hand, side-effects and toxic signs (see below) depend more on the peaks. Since there is no diurnal variation in lithium excretion, where more than one dose is given in the 24 hours the doses should be equally spaced (e.g. two, 12 hours apart, or three, 8 hours apart). This will prevent a big peak at one part of the day while providing a satisfactory basal lithium level. Another way of avoiding peaks is to prescribe sustained release tablets, which let out their lithium more slowly than ordinary tablets and so spread out and soften the peak time. But it may still be necessary to give them 12-hourly, or, more often, to split a big daily dose.

As dose follows dose, the 40 litres or so of body water become permeated by lithium ions in increasing amounts until the urinary excretion rate equals the lithium intake. The basal plasma level and body water concentration then cease to rise, and this steady state will persist for very long periods as long as the daily dose remains constant and the individual remains in health and continues to live the same regular life, eating and drinking and exercising to similar extent. An intercurrent illness, anaesthesia or surgery will change the steady state and, therefore, demand new blood tests and possibly dose change. They do not necessarily mean that lithium must be stopped, but that closer control is needed. But once a steady state is achieved there is not the same need for frequent testing that there is when beginning treatment. Provided there is no life change, once in three or six months will be enough. There are no absolute contraindications to lithium but caution is required in renal failure, heart failure, recent myocardial infarction, electrolyte imbalance, the elderly and in patients who are unreliably taking medication.

Poor renal function, as in the elderly or those with kidney disease (or even on regular renal dialysis) means more care in choosing the daily dose to be taken and more frequent monitoring of the lithium by blood tests. Patients with congestive cardiac failure with fluctuating renal function and excess variable body water, perhaps with signs of oedema, are unlikely to be suitable for lithium because of the difficulty in establishing and keeping control. The vast majority of patients to be put on lithium, however, are physically healthy.

Mechanism of action

Lithium has numerous actions on biological systems, usually at high concentrations. As the smallest alkaline cation, it can substitute for sodium, potassium, calcium and magnesium in several ways. It penetrates cells through sodium channels but is extruded less efficiently by active transport, so that the cell:plasma ratio is about 0.5 in red blood cells. Within the cell lithium interacts with systems that normally involve other cations, including transmitter release and second messenger systems. Many transmitters and hormones (including TSH, ADH at V_2 receptors, DA at D_1 receptors, and NA at beta receptors) interact with receptors that use c-AMP as the second (intracellular) messenger (see p. 27). Lithium inhibits c-AMP production in these systems. This action on ADH receptors contributes to the polyuria and polydipsia (nephrogenic diabetes insipidus), and at TSH receptors to goitre and hypothyroidism which are side-effects. Another second messenger system is the phospho-inositide cycle which controls intracellular calcium levels. This system is linked to acetylcholine muscarinic receptors, NA alpha-1, 5-HT-2, and TRH receptors, and some of these are inhibited by therapeutic levels of lithium. Lithium is thought to potentiate 5-HT responses in man although the precise mechanisms are unclear. It is also able to reduce the development of receptor super-sensitivity which occurs as a compensatory phenomenon, for instance during exposure to receptor blocking agents. It is unclear which, if any, of these actions are relevant to its therapeutic effects and neurological side-effects.

Lithium side-effects

Some side-effects occur quickly and diarrhoea and some vomiting may result from direct local tissue action. But most effects, therapeutic or otherwise, take some days to begin to appear because lithium build-up in the brain is slower than in other tissues and some of its actions involve metabolic responses. The majority of patients on lithium will experience at least one side-effect and all should be informed about side-effects and signs of toxicity. Some side-effects require an intervention and they contribute to non-adherence.

Gastrointestinal

Mild abdominal discomfort, sometimes with loose motions, may occur during the first few weeks of treatment especially with higher doses. By using divided doses these may be avoided. A slow release preparation may be better tolerated but occasionally irritates the lower bowel. Severe or persistent diarrhoea suggests toxicity. Lithium tends to reduce thyroid function. Increased TSH occurs in a quarter of patients, thyroid enlargement (goitre) in about 5%, and clinical hypothyroidism in 5–10% of patients. Those with pre-existing thyroid antibodies or a family history of thyroid disease are more likely to develop hypothyroidism. The development of hypothyroidism is often signalled by weight gain and lethargy and should be distinguished from depression. Treatment with thyroxine is usually straightforward and lithium can be continued. If lithium is withdrawn, thyroid function usually returns in about two months. Occasionally thyrotoxicosis occurs.

Kidney

Polyuria and excessive thirst with polydipsia are usually reversible but after long-term treatment are not always so. Giving lithium once daily as opposed to divided doses usually makes no difference to total daily urine volumes but may occasionally be helpful. In 1977 histological changes were reported in patients on lithium, including glomerular damage, interstitial fibrosis and tubular atrophy (focal interstitial nephropathy). Similar findings were later made in patients who had received no lithium treatment. Much further work has shown that during long-term treatment with lithium, monitored at therapeutic doses, no deterioration occurs in glomerular filtration rate in the vast majority of patients. Occasional cases of chronic renal failure have been reported and attributed by nephrologists to lithium, even in patients whose lithium levels have been monitored carefully: this is thought to be a rare idiosyncratic reaction. Episodes of lithium toxicity can produce renal damage.

Central nervous system

A fine tremor of the hands may occur and is similar to that in anxiety. It can be worsened by antidepressants.

Beta-blockers such as propranolol (starting at 10 mg, twice daily) reduce this and are best taken intermittently. Lithium can increase extrapyramidal (Parkinsonian) side-effects in patients on antipsychotic drugs, and can itself produce cogwheel rigidity in a few patients. In contrast to neuroleptic-induced Parkinsonism, this does not improve with anticholinergic drugs.

Mental and cognitive effects

Memory problems are frequent in patients interviewed about possible side-effects, but objective tests usually show little change. Some successful artists and professionals do not want to continue lithium because they sense a reduction in creativity, but the majority, although missing some hypomanic swings, consider that their long-term productivity and creativity are higher under lithium treatment.

In therapeutic doses lithium does not impair psychomotor coordination and is not a bar to driving private motor vehicles, although a diagnosis of manic–depressive illness excludes patients from driving certain public service vehicles.

Cardiovascular effects

Lithium can produce benign, reversible T-wave flattening or inversion, a pattern similar to that with hypokalaemia. Cardiac dysrhythmias are rare with therapeutic doses, especially in younger patients, but caution should be exercised when using lithium in patients with cardiac failure and the elderly.

Skin

Lithium can produce or exacerbate acne and psoriasis. Tetracyclines should be used with caution because of their possible interaction with lithium, but retinoids can be used.

Metabolic effects and weight gain

Patients tend to gain weight. The mechanism is unknown although increased consumption of sweet drinks may contribute; increased food intake and altered metabolism are also possible. Lithium produces subtle alterations in glucose and insulin metabolism and occasionally worsens control of diabetes. Fluid retention and oedema may occur with higher doses.

Parathyroid, bone and teeth

Lithium produces mild increases in parathyroid hormone level and serum calcium. No long-term effects on bone have been found in animals or adult humans. There is no direct effect of lithium upon the teeth but increased consumption of sweet drinks will lead to caries.

Sexual function

Impairment of sexual drive, arousal and ejaculation occurring in manic–depressive patients are rarely due to lithium and more likely to the underlying condition or other drugs.

Neuromuscular junction

Lithium reduces acetylcholine release and potentiates neuromuscular blocking agents including succinyl choline; it exacerbates myasthenia gravis.

Blood and bone marrow

Lithium produces a benign reversible leucocytosis, probably by an effect on marrow growth factors.

Lithium toxicity

Clinical features

Lithium toxicity is indicated by the development of three groups of symptoms – gastrointestinal, motor especially cerebellar, and cerebral. Nausea and diarrhoea progress to vomiting and incontinence. Marked fine tremor progresses to a coarse (cerebellar or Parkinsonian) tremor, giddiness, cerebellar ataxia, slurred speech, and to gross incoordination with choreiform movements and muscular twitching (myoclonus), upper motor neurone signs (spasticity and extensor plantar reflexes), electroencephalogram abnormalities and seizures. In mild toxicity there is impairment of concentration but this deteriorates into drowsiness and disorientation, and in more severe toxicity there is marked apathy and impaired consciousness leading to coma and death. Lithium toxicity can also produce myoclonus and electroencephalogram changes normally associated with Creutzfeldt-Jakob disease, but these are reversible.

Diagnosis of toxicity

Lithium toxicity should be assumed in patients on lithium with vomiting or severe nausea, cerebellar signs or disorientation. Lithium treatment should be stopped immediately, and serum lithium, urea and electrolyte levels measured. However, the severity of toxicity bears little relationship to serum lithium levels and neurotoxicity can occur with levels in the usual therapeutic range. Diagnosis should be based upon clinical judgement and not upon the blood level. Lithium should only be restarted (at an adjusted dose) when the patient's condition has improved, or an alternative cause of the symptoms has been found.

Treatment of lithium toxicity

Often cessation of lithium and provision of adequate salt and fluids, including saline infusions, will suffice. In patients with high serum levels (greater than 2 mmol/l) or coma, haemodialysis can speed the removal of lithium and reduce the risk of permanent neurological damage.

Outcome

Patients who survive episodes of lithium toxicity will often make a full recovery. However, a proportion have persistent renal or neurological damage with cerebellar symptoms, spasticity and cognitive impairment. This outcome is more likely if patients are continued on lithium while showing signs of toxicity or during intercurrent physical illnesses. The signs of toxicity develop gradually over several days during continued lithium treatment, and in some cases continue to develop for days after treatment is stopped.

Factors predisposing to lithium toxicity

Conditions of salt depletion (diarrhoea, vomiting, excessive sweating during fever or in hot climates) can lead to lithium retention. Drugs which reduce the renal excretion of lithium include thiazide diuretics (but not frusemide or amiloride), certain non-steroidal anti-inflammatory drugs (indomethacin, ibuprofen, piroxicam, naproxen, and phenylbutazone, but not aspirin, paracetamol or sulindac), and certain antibiotics (erythromycin, metronidazole and tetracycline). These drugs should be avoided if possible. If they must be used, the dose of lithium should be reduced and blood levels monitored.

In patients with serious intercurrent illnesses, especially infections, lithium should be stopped or reduced in dose and carefully monitored until the patient's condition is stable. Gastroenteritis is particularly liable to lead to toxicity.

In the elderly, renal function is decreased, lower doses of lithium are required and toxicity can develop more readily.

Uses

Lithium ('Liskonum', 'Litarex', 'Camcolit', 'Phasal', 'Priadel') may be used for:

(a)   treatment of hypomania
(b)   prevention of recurrent depression and mania, or lessening of distressing cyclothymia
(c)   treatment of irritability and aggression in the mentally handicapped
(d)   drug combination treatments of depression or schizophrenia.

Treatment of hypomania and aggression

Because it is slow to act, lithium is not the treatment of choice in manic illness, where a neuroleptic will be preferred. But is has some value in hypomanic cases because it is easy and safe to handle, and should show results within the week.

Start with 1200–1600 mg (30–40 mmol) lithium carbonate daily, divided as doses at 8 a.m. and 8 p.m., or 8 a.m., 4 p.m., midnight (smaller daily intake for the elderly, or those with poor kidney function), and take a *timed* blood sample (see introduction on lithium) at five days, and three days for the elderly. Then adjust the oral dose up or down to adjust plasma level to desired value, above 0.8 and below 1.4 mmol/l lithium.

Doses can be altered every week with monitoring blood tests. Once it is clear the right plasma level has been reached, confirm its stability on the same dose by a monthly blood test until discharge to out-patients, and then every two to three months until recovery.

Young patients may need and tolerate up to 2400 mg daily. The same procedure is appropriate for the aggressive mentally handicapped.

Prophylactic treatment of recurrent illness and other uses

In prophylaxis the effective plasma level is lower: 0.5 to 0.8 mmol/l although, occasionally, a level of 1.0 mmol/l or higher may be necessary. A daily intake of 800 mg lithium carbonate (24 mmol lithium) will be enough for most people. Again, adjust doses weekly to desired stable plasma level and, provided circumstances do not change, six-monthly follow-up tests will suffice. But make sure the patient understands about physiological and toxic signs.

If lithium is effective in prevention it will need to be continued indefinitely. Ten years without relapse is no guarantee of future health if lithium is then stopped. If it is stopped it should be by gradual reduction. Rapid bipolar cyclers (four or more attacks in the year) do not usually do very well with lithium prophylaxis and carbamazepine may be better. Where both alone have failed, combining the two may succeed.

In the treatment of depressive illness, where a tricyclic such as imipramine has failed, the addition of lithium carbonate may result in early improvement. (For use in schizophrenia see p. 104.)

Preparation of the patient

The physically healthy person requires no physical preparation beyond the routine medical history taking and physical examination. It is usual to check urea, creatinine and electrolyte levels, and to test thyroid function before commencing lithium. These provide a useful baseline. If abnormal renal function is suspected, creatinine clearance should be measured again as a baseline, but the ability to excrete lithium in the urine is best judged by the fall in plasma lithium levels with time after successive doses, rather than by creatinine clearance or blood urea. If one suspects that a patient (e.g. an elderly person) may not have good renal function, start lithium cautiously, 400 mg daily, say, and see the plasma concentration at two or five days later, adjusting the dose as before to get therapeutic levels.

Routine tests of renal, thyroid and cardiac function before and during lithium treatment in the absence of clinical evidence of disease are no substitute for the doctor clinically assessing patients in a thorough manner, looking for any sensitivity to the drug including toxic side-effects and, if present, trying to relate them to the dose schedule. When tests are done regularly, a foolproof system of noting and filing results must be devised. Too often, results go astray or float loosely in the case notes.

For physically ill people the matter is quite different, and a physician's opinion can be helpful in judging the extent of pathology.

All patients should be educated about the side-effects and signs of toxicity and given a standard information sheet by the pharmacist. They should be aware of the possibility of interactions with other drugs and of changes during illness. All doctors should be aware that it is not dangerous to discontinue lithium for a few days during an intercurrent illness or suspected toxicity.

Effects on foetus and infant

During the first three months of pregnancy, when the foetus is being formed, there is a risk of lithium producing cardiac malformations such as Ebstein's anomaly. The risk was previously thought to be as high as 10%, but a recent case control study shows it is not so. But anticonvulsants are associated with neural tube and developmental defects.

A foetus exposed to lithium in late pregnancy may be born with hypotonia and hypothyroidism; but these should clear soon. A new-born infant getting breast milk from a mother taking lithium will be receiving a lithium dose which the infantile kidney has difficulty in excreting. Hypothyroidism and goitre are the main risks to the baby.

Pregnancy in bipolar patients should, if possible, be managed without psychotropic drugs. Antipsychotics are probably the safest if antimanic medication is needed. Fortunately, pregnancy is a time of much reduced risk for recurrence of bipolar disorder, but the two weeks after childbirth are a time of greatly increased risk in a mother with a history or family history of bipolar disorder. A quarter of bipolar patients develop post-natal psychosis with manic features at this time.

Lithium and mood stabilising drugs should be stopped in pregnancy but restarted as soon as possible after childbirth. A woman who becomes pregnant while taking lithium or anticonvulsants should be counselled about the risks and offered ultra-sound screening at about 18 weeks for possible cardiac defects with a view to termination. If a woman has been taking lithium during pregnancy the dose will need to be reduced after childbirth when the glomerular filtration rate falls from a higher level back to normal.

Preparations

Lithium is available as citrate or carbonate. No injectable form is available. Liquid for oral administration can be prepared from lithium chloride or citrate.

Lithium carbonate (100 mg is 2.7 mmol Li) –
  tablets: 250 mg, 400 mg ('Camcolit')
  controlled-release tablets: 300 mg ('Phasal'), 200 mg, 400 mg ('Priadel'), 450 mg ('Liskonum')
Lithium citrate –
  controlled-release tablets: 564 mg (6 mmol Li) ('Litarex')
  liquid: 500 mg/ml 'Priadel', 520 mg/5 ml

Individuals differ in the speed with which so-called slow- or delayed-release preparations are absorbed. 'Litarex' is the only preparation which delivers reliably a slow release to the blood. However, 'Litarex' tablets are large and difficult to swallow.

Further reading

JACOBSON, S. J., JONES, K., JOHNSON, K., *et al* (1992) Prospective multicentre study of pregnancy outcome after lithium exposure during first trimester. *Lancet*, **339**, 530–533.

JOHNSON, N. (1988) *Depression and Mania: Modern Lithium Therapy.* Oxford: IRL Press.

25 Antipsychotics

These are drugs used primarily in the treatment of schizophrenia, and for mania. Some may be used as hypnotics, or in small doses against anxiety and tension. Their older name, 'neuroleptics', derives from their neurological side-effects. Chemically they form several distinct groups. The phenothiazines and the thioxanthenes resemble the tricyclics in having a three-ring structure, but the central ring has only six atoms instead of seven and one of them is sulphur: the type drugs are chlorpromazine and flupenthixol respectively. Then there are the butyrophenones (type: haloperidol) related to the analgesic pethidine, the phenylbutyl piperidines (type: pimozide), and the benzamides (type: sulpiride). More recently dibenzodiazepines (type: clozapine), and benzisoxazoles (risperidone) have been introduced.

The first effective antipsychotic, chlorpromazine, was discovered in 1952 by French workers investigating a series of antihistamines. This drug, called 'Largactil' because of its large number of pharmacological actions, was the first of a number of phenothiazines introduced into psychiatry. A few years later Janssen and colleagues investigating derivatives of pethidine in animals discovered haloperidol; noting its ability to antagonise the effects of amphetamine they studied it in schizophrenia and found it to be useful. It was introduced in 1957. The mechanism of action of the antipsychotic drugs remained unclear until 1963 when Swedish workers Carlsson and Linqvist noted increased levels of the dopamine metabolite HVA in the cerebrospinal fluid; they postulated that haloperidol and chlorpromazine blocked DA receptors (see p. 28). The receptors themselves were first identified by their binding to radioactively labelled haloperidol. It was shown that all known antipsychotics had in common the ability to bind these DA receptors and that their potency in doing so correlated highly with their potency in schizophrenia. It became widely believed that all antipsychotic effects were due to blockade of DA receptors. Drugs were then developed to be more specific in blocking DA and not other transmitters – for instance pimozide.

More recently two important developments have occurred. Firstly, DA receptors have been recognised as having subtypes (see p. 29). Blockade of D-2 receptors is thought to be important for antipsychotic effects, and the benzamide drugs, sulpiride and remoxipride, are specific D-2 antagonists. However, D-2 receptors themselves can be further subdivided, and the antipsychotics differ in the extent to which they block these different subtypes. Clozapine for instance is able to block D-4 receptors which are not blocked by haloperidol or the benzamides; some benzamides block D-3 receptors preferentially.

Secondly, the blockade of other transmitters may be important in some situations. For instance, blockade of alpha-1 and H-1 receptors may contribute to the early sedative effects and behavioural control by antipsychotics. Blockade of 5-HT-2 receptors may modify the effects of D-2 blockade, and produce a greater improvement in the symptoms of schizophrenia with less extrapyramidal side-effects, as claimed for risperidone.

Positron emission tomography scans and receptor occupancy

The technique of positron emission tomography (PET) allows the visualisation of the number and distribution of receptors in the living brain. A drug, which is selective for a particular class of receptors, is labelled with a positron emitting atom, and injected intravenously. PET then shows the distribution of the labelled drug, as it attaches to receptors in the brain. This method can be used when the patient is receiving treatment with other drugs, to determine by how much the uptake of the labelled drug is reduced; from this can be calculated the occupancy by the other drug.

In this way it has been shown that classical antipsychotics require to block 70–85% of D-2 receptors in order to treat acute schizophrenia. By contrast, clozapine occupies only about 50% of D-2 receptors, but also occupies a similar proportion of D-1 receptors, and presumably of other subtypes of DA receptors. Similarly Parkinsonian side-effects in young patients occurred only when D-2 receptor occupancy in the basal ganglia reached 75% or more.

Side-effects

DA receptors are members of the large class of receptors linked to G-proteins, and other members of the receptor class share much of the same peptide structure. It is not surprising that some drugs which block DA receptors bind also to receptors for other members of the class, in particular H-1 receptors, ACh-M, 5-HT-2, NA alpha-1 and alpha-2 receptors (see p. 27).

The side-effects of the antipsychotics can be understood in relation to their pharmacological actions. Thus blockade of DA receptors causes extrapyramidal symptoms (see Chapter 14) and neuroleptic malignant syndrome, reduced drive and hyperprolactinaemia. It probably also contributes to weight gain. Blockade of ACh-M receptors causes atropinic side-effects, dry mouth, constipation, blurred vision, urinary retention and impaired concentration; it may, however, protect against Parkinsonism, dystonia and akathisia. Blockade of alpha-1 receptors contributes to sedation and causes postural hypotension, especially in the first few days of treatment, and ejaculatory impotence. H-1 blockade produces sedation. 5-HT-1A blockade may contribute to weight gain, while 5-HT-2 blockade reduces Parkinsonism and dystonia.

Toxic and allergic reactions

Rashes may occur but are seldom a major problem. Abnormal liver function tests and cholestatic jaundice occur with phenothiazines and occasionally with haloperidol. It is prudent to assess liver function tests before and during the first two weeks of treatment. If the tests become abnormal, a switch to a different class of antipsychotic is preferable.

Agranulocytosis occurs rarely with phenothiazines, usually after 10–90 days of treatment. Frequent blood tests are of little value in detecting this, but signs of infection early in therapy should lead to an immediate full blood count.

Cardiac toxicity and sudden death

The occurrence of sudden death in patients on antipsychotics and sedative medication is currently controversial. The older literature indicated that high doses of phenothiazines, particularly thioridazine, were associated with sudden cardiovascular collapse. More recently cases have been reported involving the high-potency antipsychotics, often used in disturbed young males by injection, sometimes in high doses and in combination with a benzodiazepine. A number of mechanisms may be involved. Some patients on long-term treatment have dystonic or dyskinetic symptoms which interfere with swallowing and lead to aspiration of food and asphyxia. Other cases are unexplained. Respiratory death through laryngeal spasm and dystonia may be involved in a small number. However, the majority are probably due to cardiac dysrhythmias. Phenothiazines, especially thioridazine, and high-potency drugs such as pimozide or haloperidol in high doses can increase the QT interval and produce T-wave flattening indicative of abnormal repolarisation. This predisposes to Torsade de Pointes dysrhythmia (ventricular flutter with varying QRS complexes), and ventricular fibrillation. Factors predisposing to this development are hypokalaemia, and high levels of catecholamines, as in a patient who is struggling under restraint.

Care should be exercised in prescribing antipsychotics to patients with a history of cardiac disease, and in administering parenteral medication to control behavioural disturbance.

Pharmacokinetic interactions

The phenothiazines induce enzymes which increase their own metabolism, requiring higher doses to be given after a few weeks. Orphenadrine can also induce these enzymes. Conversely, the phenothiazines and tricyclic MARIs compete for hydroxylase enzymes in the liver, so increasing the blood levels of the tricyclics. Propranolol interferes with the metabolism of phenothiazines leading to increased blood levels. Carbamazepine induces liver enzymes and has been shown to lower blood levels of haloperidol by half within three weeks. Phenothiazines can induce phenytoin toxicity by inhibiting its metabolism.

Withdrawal effects

Abrupt withdrawal of antipsychotics may lead to nausea, agitation and insomnia and possibly to a rebound of the underlying psychosis. Those with anticholinergic properties may be more liable to withdrawal problems.

Phenothiazines

This bewilderingly large group of drugs, of which chlorpromazine was the first to be used in psychiatry, all have molecular structures on the same ground plan and broadly similar therapeutic effects, differing mainly in their side-effects (Fig. 4). The modifications to the molecule which vary the clinical effects are in the atoms attached at the asterisk-point and the side-chain 'R'. The liability to induce sleep, for instance, or Parkinsonism, is altered by changing 'R'. Particular 'R's also produce the depot phenothiazines. Attachments of fluorine atoms at the asterisk-point increases the potency of a drug. Fig. 4 will help an understanding of the inter-relations of some commonly used phenothiazines.

The drugs with the first type of (aliphatic) side-chain are low potency, and have a broad spectrum of pharmacological actions, causing sedation and hypotension but less Parkinsonism. Drugs with the second and third types of (aromatic) side-chain – the piperazines – are high potency, and produce less sedation and hypotension but more acute extrapyramidal side-effects. Thioridazine has a piperidine side-chain, and no halogen, is low potency, broad spectrum and less liable to produce Parkinsonism.

Long-acting fluphenazine decanoate ('Modecate') is made by esterifying the 'R' side-chain terminal – OH – with a long-chain fatty acid, decanoic acid, which increases its lipid solubility, and dissolving it in an oil. A single intramuscular dose may be effective for up to four weeks.

All the drugs are rapidly metabolised in the liver by oxidation of the sulphur atom in the central ring, by hydroxylation of the side-rings, and by changes in the side-chains. Most of the metabolites are clinically inactive.

Sulphoxides and hydroxy-derivatives are excreted to some extent in the urine and predominantly through the liver into the gut and then out in the faeces. The microbial flora of the gut is capable of reducing inactive sulphoxide

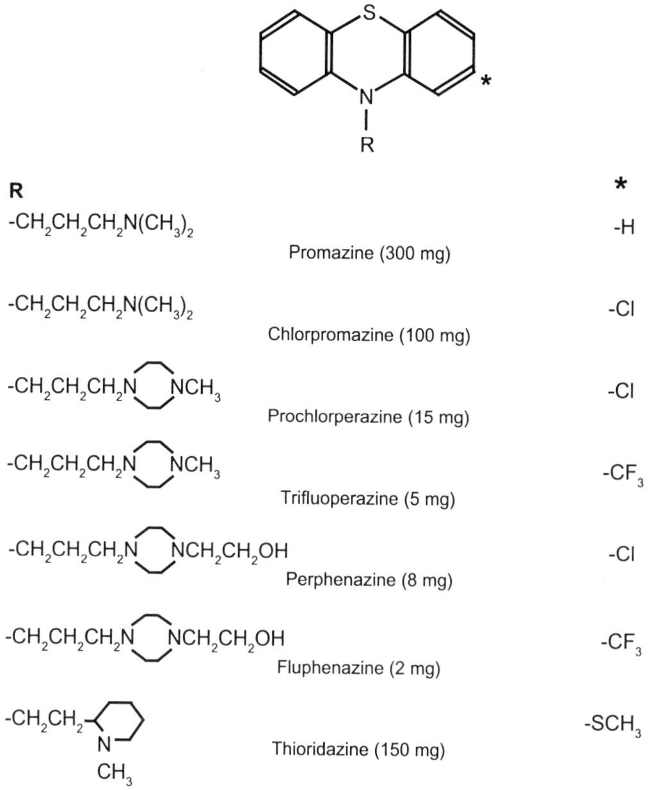

R   *

-CH$_2$CH$_2$CH$_2$N(CH$_3$)$_2$ -H

Promazine (300 mg)

-CH$_2$CH$_2$CH$_2$N(CH$_3$)$_2$ -Cl

Chlorpromazine (100 mg)

-CH$_2$CH$_2$CH$_2$N⟩ ⟨NCH$_3$ -Cl

Prochlorperazine (15 mg)

-CH$_2$CH$_2$CH$_2$N⟩ ⟨NCH$_3$ -CF$_3$

Trifluoperazine (5 mg)

-CH$_2$CH$_2$CH$_2$N⟩ ⟨NCH$_2$CH$_2$OH   -Cl

Perphenazine (8 mg)

-CH$_2$CH$_2$CH$_2$N⟩ ⟨NCH$_2$CH$_2$OH   -CF$_3$

Fluphenazine (2 mg)

-CH$_2$CH$_2$-⟩   -SCH$_3$
    N
    CH$_3$

Thioridazine (150 mg)

Fig. 4 The basic structure of phenothiazines, and roughly equivalent doses

back to the active drug which can then be reabsorbed and circulated again. Drug metabolites continue to be excreted for some months after drug-taking has stopped.

There is much variation from patient to patient in the speed of metabolism of the same drug. In some, metabolism begins in the gut wall even before absorption into the body. Metabolism is speeded up after two to three weeks of continued use. For these reasons, injected drug may be several times more effective than oral, and syrup may be more effective than tablet.

The elderly are much more sensitive to phenothiazines; therefore, use smaller doses to avoid sedation and hypotension, and use less potent drugs to avoid Parkinsonism. Normal and neurotic adults become drowsy on small doses which would not affect a schizophrenic or manic patient.

Brain-damaged patients may be unusually sensitive to phenothiazines. The tendency to have fits may be slightly increased in epilepsy, but the drugs are valuable for controlling the special irritability and aggression which sometimes occur in epilepsy.

For control of florid psychotic illnesses it is best not to be timid or tentative but to start with quite big doses – chlorpromazine 100 mg or trifluoperazine 5 mg, each thrice daily – and soon adjust the dose up or down as required. The occasional patient finds the acute dose too big and rather quickly develops a dystonic reaction, which may be misjudged as hysterical – writhing body movements, arching of the back, torticollis, protruding lolling tongue. This must be treated with anti-Parkinsonian drugs and may need an adjustment of the dose.

When one phenothiazine in full dosage as syrup or by injection has not been successful, another is unlikely to do much better. It is preferable to change to a butyrophenone or another class of antipsychotic. These are chemically quite distinct from the phenothiazines, although similar in effect. All take time, even several weeks of continuous administration to abolish schizophrenic symptoms, but are often quick to control mania.

Chlorpromazine

Chlorpromazine ('Largactil') may be used for:

(a)   control and maintenance therapy of schizophrenia and other psychoses
(b)   treatment of mania
(c)   control of the violent patient
(d)   insomnia
(e)   tension, anxiety, agitation
(f)   nausea, vomiting
(g)   appetite stimulant in anorexia nervosa.

For acutely disturbed states, chlorpromazine is the classic drug of choice (equal with haloperidol), having a prolonged quietening effect without impairment of consciousness. Chlorpromazine is therefore used to control manic states, acutely disturbed schizophrenics, delirium and confusional states, to cover drug withdrawal in the drug-dependent, and prevent outbursts in the aggressive epileptic. Large doses are tolerated and indeed required, since to gain control quickly is important.

Chlorpromazine syrup (100 mg repeated 4–6 hourly for 3–6 doses) usually achieves control; initially in the most severe, a deep intramuscular injection may be necessary, converting (by overlapping) to an oral dose as soon as cooperation is achieved. Tranquillising effects should be evident within 6–24 hours and doses of 300–800 mg a day continued. Once the abnormal behaviour is controlled, start reducing the dose.

Acute disturbance apart, chlorpromazine is invaluable for the treatment of schizophrenia, especially paranoid and catatonic types. The antipsychotic effect begins after three to six days but is more marked from two weeks, and delusions lessen, auditory hallucinations diminish or cease, and thought disorder is less marked. Start with oral chlorpromazine (150 mg daily), which may need to be raised in 150 mg daily steps, at intervals, up to 900 mg for control. Increasing the dose too quickly in the initial stages may induce hypotension or a dystonic reaction; a high dose at two to three weeks may induce Parkinsonism. Very long continued treatment causes other unwanted effects.

A dose of 25–100 mg at night produces an early hypnotic effect. Small doses (25–50 mg, three times daily) reduce nausea and vomiting, and similar doses or higher are used in anorexia nervosa to stimulate appetite and weight gain. Where minor tranquillisers might be used, 10–25 mg, three times daily, suppresses tension and anxiety in neurotic states; higher doses can lessen obsessive–compulsive symptoms.

Early side-effects

(a) Common: sedation, hypotension (dizziness), dry or nasty mouth, indigestion, blurred vision – all usually improving as soon as tolerance spontaneously develops.

(b) Uncommon: dystonia. Sudden appearance of torticollis, arching of back, tongue protrusion, writhing, abnormal movements or oculogyric crisis, all suggestive of hysterical reaction or onset of acute neurological damage. Treat by giving parenteral anticholinergic drugs. Relief begins in a few minutes. Continue with oral anticholinergics.

Medium-term side-effects

(a) Mild rash at 21 days is usually trivial, and quickly fades.

(b) Tiredness, weakness, internal restlessness (akathisia or 'jitters'), insomnia at night although drowsy by day, and Parkinsonism developing – stiffness of arms and legs, tremor, loss of facial mobility and expression, sometimes salivation. These do not spontaneously resolve. Treat with anti-Parkinsonian drugs or by reduction of phenothiazine dose.

(c) Weight gain, by degrees, of 6 kg or more to a plateau by 18 months. Reverses slowly when phenothiazine is stopped; attention to diet is advisable.

(d) Galactorrhoea can be distressing and sometimes amenorrhoea occurs. In these cases it may be possible to reduce the dose if the psychosis has improved. Reduced libido may also result from raised prolactin levels.

(e) Photosensitivity: some patients on chlorpromazine are liable to easy sunburn in summer. Avoid direct exposure (shady hats and gloves), use 'Uvistat', or other ultra-violet blocking skin cream. Consider changing to another drug which does not cause photosensitivity.

(f) Pigmentation of exposed skin, with a metallic grey–mauve colour occurs occasionally, especially in females after four years of treatment. Deposits in the cornea and lens may occur with higher doses but rarely impaired vision.

(g) Frostbite: fingers are more liable to freezing and frostbite in very cold weather, and patients should wear warm gloves when outside.

(h) Occasional epileptic fits can be treated with anticonvulsants.

(i) Jaundice: if liver function tests deteriorate, or cholestatic jaundice develops, chlorpromazine should be stopped. Treatment should be resumed later with a different drug.

(j) When continued in large doses in patients with constipation, perforation of the bowel may occur as a result of ischaemic necrosis.

(k) Agranulocytosis occurs rarely.

Late side-effects: tardive dyskinesia

After a year or more of continuous drug treatment, especially in the elderly or where there is brain damage (neurological disease, head injury, dementia) abnormal, involuntary movements appear, especially around the mouth and tongue (see p. 137).

Contraindications and interactions

Chlorpromazine is compatible with all drugs and with electroconvulsive therapy.

Chlorpromazine stimulates liver drug metabolism after about two weeks of use. The increased rate of metabolism declines in about two weeks on stopping phenothiazines.

Chlorpromazine blocks the liver metabolism of some drugs, such as morphine, pethidine, and tricyclic antidepressants, increasing blood levels.

Chlorpromazine is contraindicated where the patient is already semi-comatose from barbiturates or alcohol, or is known to suffer from liver disease such as cirrhosis, or immediately following an attack of hepatitis. Where there is a history of a previous allergic response to chlorpromazine, it will be better to try a different phenothiazine, for example trifluoperazine. Large doses may diminish symptoms of acute abdomen and of fevers, making physical diagnosis harder.

Preparations

Tablets: 10 mg, 25 mg, 50 mg, 100 mg
Syrup: 25 mg per 5 ml
Forte suspension: 100 mg per 5 ml
Injection (intramuscular): 25 mg per ml in 1 ml and 2 ml ampoules.
Suppositories: 100 mg

Thioridazine

Thioridazine ('Melleril') is particularly useful in calming agitation and restlessness but otherwise is used for the same purposes as chlorpromazine, although there is no injectable form. For control of psychosis, a dose one and a half times that of chlorpromazine is used. It is used in the elderly because, of all phenothiazines, it is the least likely to produce extrapyramidal signs, having pronounced anticholinergic properties. Dizziness and muzziness resulting from hypotension, especially postural hypotension, may occur particularly at the start of treatment. Either use smaller doses, raise the dose more gradually, or change to another phenothiazine. Doses above 600 mg a day, particularly for longer than four weeks, must be avoided as they carry the risk of pigmentary retinopathy and blindness.

Preparations

Tablets: 10 mg, 25 mg, 50 mg, 100 mg
Syrup: 25 mg per 5 ml
Suspension: 25 mg and 100 mg per 5 ml

Promazine

Promazine ('Sparine') is much less potent as an antipsychotic than chlorpromazine; it is used as a hypnotic or sedative for the elderly where drug-induced confusional states are a risk. Beware of producing over-sedation, urinary and faecal incontinence, disorientation, and lowered temperature.

Orally give 25–100 mg once, or up to four times daily; intramuscularly give 50 mg, repeatable after six hours.

Preparations

Suspension: 50 mg per 5 ml
Injection: 50 mg per ml in 1 ml and 2 ml ampoules

Trifluoperazine

Trifluoperazine ('Stelazine') is much more potent than chlorpromazine; it produces little sedation or hypotension but is more liable to produce dystonia, akathisia and Parkinsonism. It is more suitable for the less behaviourally disturbed patient, for instance out-patients.

For paranoid psychosis and schizophrenia give 10–30 mg daily by mouth, in divided doses, or as a spansule at night. Give 1–5 mg once or more daily for symptomatic anxiety. Do not prescribe anti-Parkinsonian drugs as a routine, but warn patients of the possible need and be ready to give them at once if they are needed. Review the question of need at two, four and eight weeks continuous treatment, since the need may disappear as the psychosis settles, or if the phenothiazine dose is reduced for maintenance treatment.

Preparations

Tablets: 1 mg, 5 mg
Spansules: 2 mg, 10 mg, 15 mg
Syrup: 1 mg per 5 ml
Concentrate: 10 mg per ml
Injection: 1 mg per ml, in 1 ml ampoules

Perphenazine

The use and side-effects of perphenazine ('Fentazin') are as for chlorpromazine, but it is less sedative and more prone to Parkinsonism.

Give 4–8 mg thrice daily as tablets, or 10 mg by intramuscular injection, and then repeating 5 mg six-hourly.

For anxiety, give 2 mg twice or thrice daily, and upwards. Has been successfully used for intractable hiccough.

Preparations

Tablets: 2 mg, 4 mg, 8 mg
Liquid concentrate: 2 mg/ml
Injection: 5 mg per 1 ml ampoule

Pericyazine

Pericyazine ('Neulactil') is used for treating psychoses and behavioural disturbance, in doses of 15–30 mg by mouth for psychoses, but up to 300 mg daily for severe behavioural disturbance due to psychosis or mental handicap.

Side-effects are as for chlorpromazine but pericyazine is more sedative.

Preparations

Tablets: 2.5 mg, 10 mg, 25 mg
Syrup: 10 mg/5 ml

Related phenothiazines

Methotrimeprazine ('Noxinan') –
    tablets: 25 mg (maximum daily dose 200 mg)
    injection: 25 mg/ml
Prochlorperazine ('Stemetil') –
    tablets: 5 mg, 25 mg (maximum daily dose 100 mg)
    syrup: 5 mg/5 ml
    granules: 5 mg in sachet

Fluphenazine and its decanoate

Fluphenazine hydrochloride ('Moditen', 'Prolixen') is the most potent of the phenothiazines. Fluphenazine decanoate ('Modecate') is fluphenazine esterified in the side-chain with decanoic acid, a long-chain fatty acid, and dissolved in sesame oil with benzyl alcohol, for injection. A single dose will continue to give therapeutic benefit for one to six weeks. The drug is injected into a muscle where it remains as a fatty depot; from this depot the drug is gradually removed via the lymphatic system, including the action of phagocytes, and the active drug is released. The injection is eminently suitable for long-term treatment of chronic schizophrenia, particularly in out-patients who may not be able, or willing, particularly if they feel well, to take tablets regularly for very long periods, or for patients suspicious of tablets. It is also useful in preventing frequently recurrent attacks of mania or hypomania.

Fluphenazine need only be taken orally once a day in a dose of 1–10 mg. At least 5 mg is required to treat a psychosis. There is considerable individual variation in absorption of the drug.

'Modecate' is given by deep intramuscular injection into the gluteal muscle. When starting depot treatment, a test dose of 12.5 mg (6.25 mg in the elderly) is given, to detect any allergic response to the vehicle and to familiarise the patient with the drug. Three to seven days later the patient starts on a regular dose of 25–50 mg weekly which continues for four to six weeks during which time previous oral medication is gradually withdrawn. The maintenance dose of 'Modecate' varies for individuals; between 6.25 mg and 100 mg given every two to six weeks. Lower doses are required in females, with increasing age, and with longer periods since the last relapse. The most common dose is 25 mg a fortnight, or the equivalent. Dystonic reactions, tremor and restlessness may occur in the two days after the injection, as a portion of free fluphenazine is released from the depot. During this time the patient may need anticholinergic medication. Some patients continue to experience such side-effects throughout the course of the injections and need to continue on anticholinergic drugs. Side-effects can sometimes be avoided by halving the dose and giving the injection twice as often. Minor degrees of side-effects, especially drowsiness or flatness, and restlessness, are not uncommon and it may take some months for the patient to adjust to them.

Sometimes, in otherwise well-controlled patients, symptoms begin to reappear towards the end of the third or fourth week after the injection; this is a sign to shorten the interval between injections or to increase the dose a little. The aim is to find the optimal interval and the smallest dose which will achieve control.

After a relapse has been brought under control it is possible to reduce the dose over the following six months. After that, if the patient is stable, the dose may be reduced to one which has previously been found to maintain the patient's stability. If it is known that a patient has previously relapsed when the dose is reduced below a certain level, then they should be advised to continue on that dose or higher. When planning a reduction of dose with the patient, remember that for pharmacokinetic reasons the full effect of the reduction will not occur until four to six months after the prescription is changed, and there is an increased risk of relapse for up to two years. Most will do well on 25 mg fortnightly; some manage on even less.

Patients feel better on lower doses, have less Parkinsonism and less risk of tardive dyskinesia. The patient should therefore be regularly and not too infrequently supervised. This can be done if the injection is administered by a community psychiatric nurse who arranges for the patient to be reviewed by the doctor. Even the most stable patient should be reviewed at least once a year and the review should preferably include a doctor who knows the patient. Team reviews or 'community ward rounds' enable information to be shared and experience to be gained.

Preparations

Fluphenazine hydrochloride ('Moditen') –
  tablets: 1 mg, 2.5 mg, 5 mg
Fluphenazine decanoate ('Modecate') –
  injection (25 mg/ml): 0.5 ml, 1.0 ml, 2.0 ml ampoules
  ready-filled disposable 1.0 ml and 2.0 ml syringes
Fluphenazine decanoate ('Modecate' concentrate)
  injection (100 mg/ml): 0.5 ml, 1.0 ml ampoules

Thioxanthenes

Thioxanthenes resemble phenothiazines closely, but have a carbon atom in place of the nitrogen atom of the middle ring to which the side-chain is attached. The side-chain is usually linked to this carbon by a double bond, which makes the molecule look a little like a tricyclic antidepressant with a sulphur atom (but a six- not a seven-atom central ring). The thioxanthene analogue of chlorpromazine is chlorprothixene ('Taractan'); flupenthixol is the analogue of fluphenazine, while zuclopenthixol has a chlorine atom, as does chlorprothixene, but a side-chain like flupenthixol. Both are available as decanoates for depot injection. The thioxanthenes are pharmacologically different from phenothiazines in that they block both D-1 and D-2 receptor types (Fig. 5).

Flupenthixol

By deep intramuscular injection, flupenthixol decanoate ('Depixol') is effective against schizophrenic symptoms (20–100 mg every two to four weeks), comparable with 'Modecate' but less sedative. It tends to be preferred in the more lethargic patient or one with a history of depression. Begin with a test intramuscular dose of 20 mg. Rarely, doses can go up to 400 mg weekly. The long-acting injection may also be tried to control mania when other treatments have failed (40–80 mg weekly), and continued, to prevent relapse. Like other major tranquillisers, oral flupenthixol ('Fluanxol') can be given in smaller doses (0.5–1.5 mg, morning and midday) for anxiety, and the higher dose tablet ('Depixol') used to suppress a psychosis (3–9 mg, twice daily).

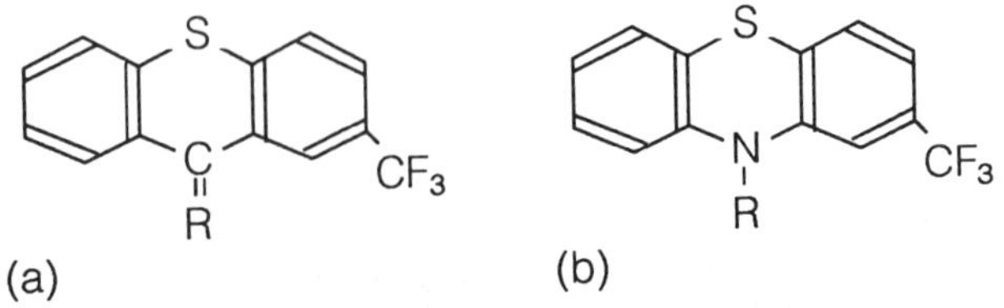

Fig. 5   Thioxanthene and phenothiazine compared: (a) flupenthixol; (b) fluphenazine

A few patients become overactive, and low doses are sometimes used as an antidepressant (see p. 77).

Preparations

Flupenthixol –
   tablets: 'Fluanxol' 0.5 mg, 1 mg
            'Depixol' 3 mg
Flupenthixol decanoate ('Depixol') –
   2% ampoules (clear): 20 mg in 1 ml, 40 mg in 2 ml
   10% ampoules (amber): 100 mg in 1 ml
   20% ampoules (amber): 200 mg in 1 ml

Zuclopenthixol

Zuclopenthixol ('Clopixol') is more sedative than flupenthixol and is more suitable for the behaviourally disturbed patient. Oral doses begin with 20–50 mg daily to a maximum of 150 mg daily. Acutely disturbed patients who consistently refuse oral medication may be given zuclopenthixol acetate ('Acuphase') by deep intramuscular injection with a duration of three days. Start with 50–150 mg, repeated after one to three days to a maximum of 400 mg in total. Zuclopenthixol decanoate can be used to follow this or for longer-term treatment; start with 100 mg intramuscular gluteal injection, and increase up to 200–500 mg every one to four weeks. The maximum dose is 600 mg a week.

Preparations

Zuclopenthixol Di HCl (oral)
   tablets: 2 mg, 10 mg, 25 mg
Zuclopenthixol decanoate ('Clopixol')
   injection (200 mg/ml): 1.0 ml ampoule, 10 ml vial
   injection (500 mg/ml): 1.0 ml ampoule with needle
Zuclopenthixol acetate ('Acuphase')
   injection (50 mg/ml): 1 ml, 2 ml ampoules

Butyrophenones and butylpiperidines

These drugs, related chemically to the analgesic pethidine, are mostly used in psychiatry for the control of schizophrenia, mania and acute brain syndrome, especially when aggression and excitement are present. Haloperidol blocks DA D-2 receptors, and to a lesser extent NA alpha-1 receptors. Pimozide is more selective for DA receptors, and less sedative. Although chemically quite distinct from phenothiazines, their therapeutic effects are similar, but some individual patients may do better with one type of drug than with the other. Some are long-acting, presumably because they are slowly metabolised and excreted, for instance pimozide (see Fig. 6 – The structure of haloperidol).

Haloperidol

Haloperidol ('Serenace', 'Haldol') may be used for:

(a)   severe excitement, overactivity or aggression, especially associated with mania or schizophrenia

(b)   continuous treatment of mania, schizophrenia and paranoid psychosis

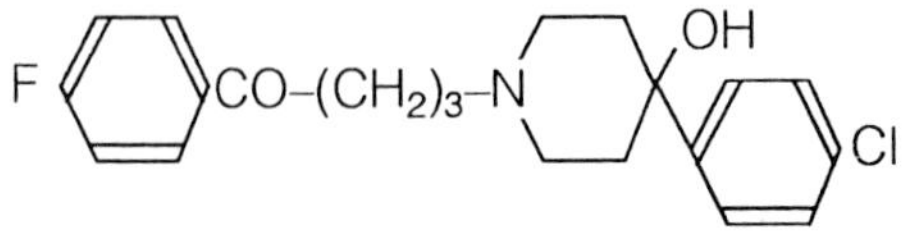

Fig. 6   The structure of haloperidol

(c)   restlessness and agitation in the elderly
(d)   acute confusional states (see p. 129)
(e)   Gilles de la Tourette's syndrome.

For the acutely excited and overactive patient, begin with 5–10 mg intramuscularly, repeated two-hourly, up to 60 mg total over 12 hours if necessary. This dosage controls most states, and when it does the dose can be reduced to 5–10 mg thrice daily orally and then further reduced in a few days depending on the response. Because of the side-effects, oral procyclidine (10 mg, thrice daily) may need to be given. If intravenous haloperidol is given, then intravenous procyclidine (5 mg) may be given at the same time but in a separate syringe. These high doses of haloperidol are required in manic, drug-induced, and schizophrenic excitements, but lower doses may be quite adequate for acute brain syndromes.

In continued treatment for mania and schizophrenia, 3–5 mg thrice daily is usually adequate, but a frequent check for psychotic symptoms and side-effects should guide. For some schizophrenics, larger doses may be needed and may be well tolerated. Claims are made that doses up to 80 mg a day are effective in resistant cases, but this is not yet accepted practice, or proven. More often the drug is now used in depot form for maintenance therapy.

For agitation in the elderly give 0.5 mg, twice daily. Children with Gilles de la Tourette's syndrome should be maintained on the lowest effective dose, which is likely to be around 0.1 mg/kg a day. Pimozide (see below) is a good alternative (0.05–0.20 mg/kg).

Side-effects

Extrapyramidal effects are common, more so than with chlorpromazine, and can come on at any stage of treatment. Stiffness, rigidity or extreme restlessness are the most frequent. The elderly and those with basal ganglia disease are especially prone to these.

Side-effects can occur with remarkable suddenness even after a single small dose, although more likely with larger doses. They may appear as excitement lessens. Side-effects may persist for three months or longer after stopping haloperidol. Intravenous procyclidine (10 mg) relieves acute symptoms. Oral anti-Parkinsonian drugs are given only when side-effects appear. Test at intervals, by their gradual withdrawal, whether they continue to be needed during long-term treatment.

Haloperidol decanoate is used similarly to fluphenazine decanoate with intervals of up to four to six weeks, but with twice the dose. Start with a test dose of 50 mg deeply intramuscular, followed by 100–200 mg, two- to four-weekly, depending on the urgency to control symptoms. Maintenance doses of 100–300 mg four-weekly are usual.

Preparations

Tablets: 1.5 mg, 5 mg, 10 mg, 20 mg
Capsules: 0.5 mg
Liquid: 2 mg per ml, 10 mg per ml
Injection: 5 mg in 1 ml, 10 mg in 1 ml, 20 mg in 2 ml

Haloperidol decanoate in oil –
    ampoules: 50 mg in 1 ml; 100 ml in 1 ml

Related drugs

Trifluoperidol ('Triperidol') –
    tablets: 0.5 and 1 mg (maximum daily dose 8 mg)
Benperidol ('Anquil') (see p. 310) –
    tablets: 0.25 mg (maximum daily dose 1.5 mg)
Droperidol ('Droleptan') –
    tablets: 10 mg
    liquid: 1 mg/ml
    injection: 5 mg/ml in 2 ml ampoule
    Use as for haloperidol and in similar dosage.

Pimoxide

Pimozide ('Orap') may be used for:

(a)   schizophrenia and paranoid psychosis
(b)   mania
(c)   Gilles de la Tourette's syndrome
(d)   monosymptomatic delusional hypochondriasis.

It has a long duration of action with a half-life averaging 53 hours, and does accumulate during regular doses.

An electrocardiogram should be done before starting treatment and in those on more than 16 mg daily. Pimozide is contraindicated if there is any history of cardiac arrhythmia or a prolonged QT interval. It is more potent than other antipsychotics as a calcium antagonist. Other drugs that prolong the QT interval should be avoided in combination, for instance tricyclic antidepressants and other antipsychotics.

For acute psychosis it is given once daily in a starting dose of 10 mg which can be increased by weekly steps of 2 or 4 mg to a maximum of 20 mg. For other indications start with 2 mg and increase gradually by 2 mg steps to a maximum of 16 mg. Its advantages are that it is fairly free of sedative and hypotensive side-effects. Parkinsonism, dystonia and akathisia may occur and require treatment. Its long half-life means that its plasma concentration changes rather slowly, and even missing a day's dose will not alter the level much.

In monosymptomatic delusional hypochondriasis, for instance delusional parasitosis, it has some unique benefits. The dose should start at 2 mg daily, increasing to 16 mg.

For children with Gilles de la Tourette's, give 0.05–0.20 mg/kg per day.

Preparations

Tablets: 2 mg, 4 mg, 10 mg

Fluspirilene

Fluspirilene ('Redeptin') is an injectable phenylbutyl piperidine suspension, with a duration of up to two weeks. Local fibrotic nodules tend to develop at the injection sites.

Preparations

Solution: 2 mg/ml in 1 ml, 2 ml ampoules, 6 ml vial

Oxypertine

Oxypertine ('Integrin') is used as an adjunct in the treatment of psychosis, especially for acute agitation or behavioural disturbance. Start with 80 mg daily, rising to a maximum of 300 mg. The drug can bring about the release of catecholamines, as reserpine. Combined use with MAOIs should be avoided. Low doses may produce agitation and hyperactivity but higher doses are sedative.

Preparations

Capsules: 10 mg
Tablets: 40 mg

Doses of depot injections

It is impossible to generalise about the equivalent doses of drugs in individuals whose metabolism varies. The depot formulations are less affected by metabolic differences, and the following are approximately equivalent when given at the same intervals: fluphenazine decanoate (25 mg); haloperidol decanoate (50 mg); pipothiazine palmitate (25 mg); flupenthixol decanoate (40 mg); zuclopenthixol decanoate

(200 mg). The last two have shorter durations and need to be given more often. In the elderly different doses apply for each drug.

Atypical antipsychotics

This term is used to describe antipsychotic drugs which are relatively lacking in extrapyramidal side-effects.

Sulpiride

Sulpiride ('Dolmatil', 'Sulpitil') is a benzamide and is selective for D-2 receptors, including the D-3 subtype. At low doses it has activating effects thought to be due to blockade of presynaptic DA auto-receptors. It is particularly potent in blocking DA receptors in the pituitary and increasing prolactin levels. It has also been used as an antidepressant. Its activating effect is not specific for depression or schizophrenia. At the higher doses needed to suppress positive symptoms, the activating effect is lost. Higher doses have also been found effective in mania (Fig. 7).

It is not metabolised to any extent but excreted unchanged in the urine. Parkinsonism, if it occurs, is mild. Anticholinergic side-effects are minimal and tardive dyskinesia so far rare. Poisoning by overdose can mean restlessness and clouding of consciousness, leading on to coma and low blood pressure; but there have been no deaths and recovery is quick.

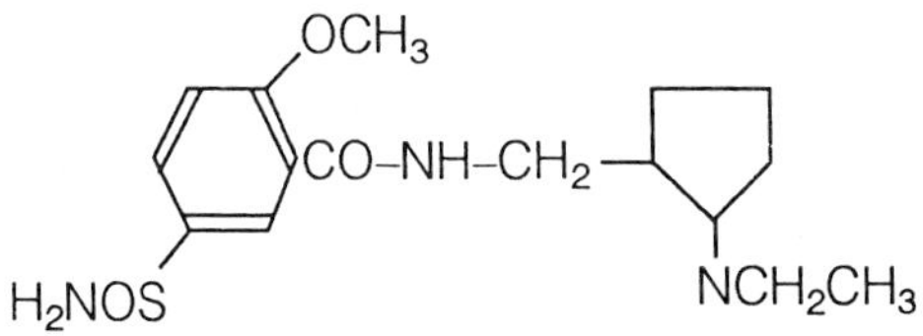

Fig. 7   The structure of sulpiride

For positive schizophrenic symptoms, start with 400 mg, twice daily, rising quickly to a maximum of 1200 mg, twice daily. For negative symptoms try reducing the dose of 400 mg towards 200 mg, twice daily. In general, do not change dose more often than once per week.

Preparations

Tablets: 200 mg

Remoxipride

Remoxipride ('Roxiam') is a benzamide which is also a selective D-2 antagonist although, like haloperidol, it also blocks sigma receptors which are of unknown function. It is as effective as haloperidol in schizophrenia but produces less extrapyramidal side-effects, probably because it binds to a subtype of D-2 receptors in the limbic system to a greater extent than those in the basal ganglia. It is also less potent than haloperidol on pituitary D-2 receptors, so produces less rise in prolactin. It has not been found effective in mania. Only an oral form is available.

It is particularly suitable for those schizophrenics who will adhere to oral medication, and who do not need sedation, and for those troubled by acute extrapyramidal side-effects with other drugs. Start with 300 mg daily, as extended release tablets, and adjust to 150–450 mg daily. The maximum dose is 600 mg.

Side-effects include tiredness, restlessness and weight gain.

It is metabolised partly by liver hydroxylation and it can induce liver enzymes.

Unlike sulpiride it is not claimed to have activating or antidepressant effects at low doses.

Note: Because several cases of aplastic anaemia have occurred in patients on remoxipride, it should not be given to those with a history of blood dyscrasia. Special care should be taken with patients previously treated with clozapine or carbamazepine which may affect the blood count. Patients starting on remoxipride should have a full blood count before starting treatment, one weekly for six months, and monthly thereafter. They should be warned to report bruising, bleeding, fever, sore throat or signs of infection. If there is evidence of an abnormality in their blood count, remoxipride should be stopped and the patient referred to a specialist haematologist.

Preparations

Capsules (extended release): 150 mg, 300 mg

Clozapine

Clozapine ('Clozaril') is a dibenzodiazepine and carries a risk of agranulocytosis in about 3% of those who take it. However, it is useful in schizophrenics who have shown resistance to other antipsychotics. It also produces less acute extrapyramidal side-effects and can lead to improvement in severe tardive dyskinesia.

It can only be used orally and the patient must agree to weekly blood counts for 18 weeks, then every two weeks as long as treatment continues. Treatment is monitored by the "Clozaril Patient Monitoring Service" (Sandoz; telephone 0276-692255), with which the doctor must register before the pharmacy can dispense.

It has a very broad spectrum of pharmacological activity at class II receptors (see p. 27), blocking all types of DA receptor (D1–5), including some (D-4) that are not blocked by other antipsychotics, H-1, ACh-M, NA alpha-1 and alpha-2, and a potent action at 5-HT-2 receptors. Side-effects are marked and include sedation, hypotension, nausea, vomiting and fits. Although atropinic side-effects occur, it commonly produces hypersalivation; this may need the addition of another anticholinergic drug. Weight gain occurs and neuroleptic malignant syndrome has been recorded. Parkinsonian symptoms are generally mild and the risk of tardive dyskinesia is lower than with other drugs. The rise in prolactin levels is also much smaller.

Patients selected for treatment should have had an unsatisfactory improvement despite the use of adequate doses of at least two other antipsychotics prescribed for sufficient duration; also those who had severe neurological side-effects limiting the use of other antipsychotic drugs. Before treatment, which starts as an in-patient, the patient should have a full blood count. The starting dose is 25 mg daily increasing by 25–50 mg daily to 300 mg daily within two weeks or longer. This gradual increase helps to reduce the incidence of intolerable side-effects. The dose is then adjusted to between 200–450 mg per day in most cases with a maximum of 900 mg per day. If treatment is stopped it should be done gradually because of the risk of rebound exacerbation of psychosis which will be difficult to control with other antipsychotics.

Patients should be reminded to report if they develop an infection, fever or sore throat so that a full blood count may be done immediately.

Concurrent use of other drugs should be avoided, especially those affecting the bone marrow and including depot antipsychotics because of their long duration. If necessary, haloperidol may be added or continued.

So far about 3% of patients treated have developed neutropenia and had their treatment stopped; 0.6% of patients developed agranulocytosis. These occurred mostly at between 4–20 weeks of starting treatment.

Improvement continues to develop for up to one year, but most improvement occurs in the first 12 weeks, and patients should not continue treatment beyond four to six months if there is no response. About 50% of patients benefit. Paranoid patients seem to benefit most, as do those with an onset after the age of 20. Both positive and negative symptoms improve along with social functioning.

The improvement in severe tardive dyskinesia begins within the first few months and continues for three years.

Preparations

Tablets: 25 mg, 100 mg

Loxapine

Loxapine ('Loxapac') is a dibenzoxapine antipsychotic, with risks of dystonia, Parkinsonism, epileptic fits, hypotension and drowsiness. It does not have the advantages of clozapine, although structurally similar.

Dose 10 mg twice daily, rising over 10 days to a daily total of 80–100 mg.

Preparations

Capsules: 10 mg, 25 mg, 50 mg

Risperidone

Risperidone ('Risperdal') is a benzisoxazole. It resembles clozapine in that it is a potent 5-HT-2 and D-2 antagonist. It also blocks H-1, NA alpha-1 and alpha-2, but not ACh or D-1 receptors. It is effective in schizophrenia, with a low incidence of extrapyramidal symptoms. In chronic schizophrenics with persistent symptoms it may provide a greater improvement in positive symptoms, negative symptoms and depression than older antipsychotics. However, these advantages are limited to a narrow range of doses, 4–8 mg daily. It is therefore suitable for schizophrenics who are maintained on modest doses of other antipsychotics but have persistent symptoms or Parkinsonism.

Side-effects of sedation and hypotension can be avoided by increasing the dose gradually. Weight gain occurs and occasionally impairment of ejaculation or orgasm. It blocks D-2 receptors in the pituitary and increases prolactin levels.

Treatment starts with 1 mg, twice daily, increasing to 2 mg, twice daily, and 3 mg, twice daily, on the next two days. The optimal dose is 2–4 mg twice daily. Doses above 10 mg daily confer no added benefit but increase the occurrence of extrapyramidal side-effects, and doses above 16 mg a day should not be used.

The drug is metabolised partly by liver hydroxylase and has an active metabolite with similar properties. The combined half-life is about 24 hours.

Preparations

Tablets: 1 mg, 2 mg, 3 mg, 4 mg

Further reading

FARDE, L., NORDSTOM, A. L., WIESEL, F. A., *et al* (1992) Positron emission tomographic analysis of central D-1 and D-2 dopamine receptor occupancy in patients treated with classical neuroleptics and clozapine. *Archives of General Psychiatry*, **49**, 538–544.

LIEBERMAN, J. A., SALTZ, B. L., JOHNS, C. A., *et al* (1991) The effects of clozapine on tardive dyskinesia. *British Journal of Psychiatry*, **158**, 503–510.

26 Anti-Parkinsonian drugs

Extrapyramidal symptoms encountered in psychiatric practice are nearly all drug-induced (see p. 135 – Extrapyramidal reactions). Only a small number result from primary basal ganglia disease, although the ageing or damaged brain is predisposed to Parkinsonian side-effects and tardive dyskinesia. Phenothiazines with a piperazine side-chain ('R' in Fig. 4, p. 239, e.g. trifluoperazine) and the butyrophenones are the two groups of antipsychotic drugs that most commonly cause Parkinsonism and other extrapyramidal syndromes. On occasion, tricyclic antidepressants in high doses may also be responsible; with lower doses, adding lithium will also provoke such reactions.

Parkinson's disease itself was first successfully treated with the atropine group of drugs which block cholinergic activity. Subsequently atropine-like synthetic drugs, also antihistaminic in action, were developed, and then drugs which increased the effectiveness of natural basal ganglia dopamine, such as L-dopa, bromocriptine and amantidine. Neither of these latter drugs is useful in drug-induced Parkinsonism, but they are relevant to psychiatric practice because of their side-effects or their occasional use for primary Parkinsonism in psychiatric patients.

Fifteen per cent of patients taking L-dopa develop significant psychiatric symptoms and may present to the psychiatrist with a toxic confusional state (acute brain syndrome), depression, hypomania, or paranoid state; L-dopa has then to be reduced or stopped. Dopamine agonists such as bromocriptine can produce psychotic reactions. Amantidine is less of a problem but in a few patients, especially those who have had a previous psychiatric illness, psychotic states with confusion and hallucinations can occur.

The synthetic anti-cholinergic drugs, procyclidine, benztropine and benzhexol, and more sedative ones such as orphenadrine, can control or modify drug-induced extrapyramidal disorders so that antipsychotic medication may be maintained. Anti-Parkinsonian drugs should not be prescribed routinely to patients on antipsychotic drugs, only when side-effects appear. The psychotropic action of phenothiazines may be modified and the early stages of tardive dyskinesia masked by anti-Parkinsonian drugs. If extrapyramidal symptoms do appear, consider reducing the level of antipsychotic drug before prescribing anti-Parkinsonian drugs long term.

Anticholinergic drugs

These block ACh-M receptors. In the caudate putamen, DA normally acts to inhibit ACh neurones. Most antipsychotic drugs block this action of DA, and thereby increase release of ACh. In addition to their antimuscarinic or 'atropinic' actions, the drugs are also to varied extents anti-histaminic, and block DA-reuptake. The latter causes stimulant effects and a risk of abuse and dependence. High doses cause confusional states or psychotic reactions.

The synthetic anticholinergic drugs used in large doses, especially in the elderly, can produce an acute brain syndrome. Their anticholinergic activity can interfere with the treatment of glaucoma, and provoke acute retention of urine in men with prostatic hypertrophy. Side-effects may appear before the optimal dose for controlling Parkinsonian symptoms is achieved. Procyclidine is discussed in some detail as the type drug, and others described briefly. Despite similar action, one of these drugs may suit a patient better than others; be prepared, if side-effects develop, to try an alternative.

Procyclidine

Procyclidine ('Arpicolin', 'Kemadrin') is widely used to relieve drug-induced, extrapyramidal symptoms and is administered intravenously to relieve acute dystonia. The drug is well absorbed from the gut and is metabolised rapidly. Intravenous or intramuscular procyclidine, usually 10 mg, relieves acute dystonia within 5–10 minutes and gives relief for 30 minutes to 4 hours. The half-life is 12 hours and often oral doses, twice daily, are enough.

When beginning neuroleptic medication, try to do without anti-muscarinic drugs until side-effects show; then start with procyclidine (5 mg, twice daily), gradually increasing every two to three doses up to 5–10 mg, three times daily. Once the side-effects are controlled, try to slowly reduce the drug every three to four months and, if possible, withdraw medication. Alternatively, the neuroleptic may be able to be reduced to a level with fewer side-effects.

An acutely disturbed patient can need very high doses of neuroleptics quickly, and then giving concurrent procyclidine avoids potential additional stress from painful side-effects. It also can help with later compliance.

Side-effects, typical of all anti-muscarinic drugs, include drowsiness, dry mouth, blurred vision, dilated pupils, nausea and constipation. Higher doses, especially in the elderly, can cause confusion and hallucinations. Avoid their use in glaucoma or prostatic hypertrophy as an acute obstruction can occur. Sound rules are to keep to the lowest dose possible to relieve extrapyramidal symptoms and, if changing dose, do it gradually. Sudden stoppage can produce acute side-effects (akinesia, rigidity, salivation, urinary retention).

Some patients experience a pleasurable 'buzz' with procyclidine and hoard or trade tablets with others to get a large supply. Higher doses produce euphoria and, rarely, hallucinations. A useful sign is fixed dilated pupils.

Preparations

Tablets: 5 mg
Syrup: 2.5 mg/5 ml; 5 mg/5 ml
Injection: 5 mg/ml

Benzhexol

Benzhexol ('Artane', 'Broflex') is used similarly to procyclidine. Start with a low dose, 1 mg daily, and increase slowly, allowing two to three days to elapse between each increase. An effective dose is usually between 5–15 mg daily. It has more pronounced stimulant effects than procyclidine and is more prone to abuse. Higher doses may well precipitate an excited and abnormal mental state; then try another drug.

Preparations

Tablets: 2 mg, 5 mg
Syrup: 5 mg/5 ml

Benztropine

Benztropine ('Cogentin') is more sedative and more slowly excreted and so is cumulative. Start with a low dose (0.5 mg) once daily for the first few days and increase gradually to 6 mg daily, if necessary. Some patients do better on divided doses, some on a single, daily dose. Acute dystonic reactions are relieved by 2 mg given intramuscularly or intravenously.

Preparations

Tablets: 2 mg
Injection: 1 mg/ml

Orphenadrine

Orphenadrine ('Biorphen', 'Disipal') is usually well tolerated by patients and is less prone to abuse than benzhexol or procyclidine. Start with 50 mg, three times daily, and increase, if necessary, up to 200 mg daily. Large overdoses may be fatal.

Preparations

Tablets: 50 mg
Elixir: 25 mg/5 ml

Biperiden

Biperiden ('Akineton') is similar to, but more sedative than, orphenadrine. Start with 1 mg, twice daily, and increase up to 6–12 mg daily. The parenteral preparation may cause hypotension; if administered intravenously, give slowly and as a dosage of 2.5–5.0 mg.

Preparations

Tablets: 2 mg
Injection: 5 mg/ml

Tetrabenazine

Tetrabenazine ('Nitoman') is used for the control of abnormal movement disorders such as Huntington's chorea and tardive dyskinesia. It works by depleting neuronal stores of biogenic amines including DA; this is similar to the action of reserpine but less pronounced. Start with 25 mg daily and gradually increase to 25 mg, three times daily, up to a maximum of 200 mg daily. If there is no improvement after seven days of high-dose treatment, do not persist with the drug. Drowsiness, indigestion, hypotension, and Parkinsonism occur as side-effects at high doses. If depression occurs, an MARI antidepressant may be given; MAOIs must be avoided because of the risk of a confusional state.

Preparation

Tablets: 25 mg

27 Anti-anxiety drugs and hypnotics

Benzodiazepines

Benzodiazepines are valuable hypnotics, anxiolytics or 'minor tranquillisers', and anticonvulsants. It is difficult to commit suicide with them in overdose when they alone are taken, and they can safely be taken with other drugs without serious interactions.

All benzodiazepines work mainly by increasing GABA transmission in the central nervous system (CNS), but CNS tolerance develops within days or weeks. The biochemical mechanism is unknown but dependence develops and unpleasant symptoms occur on withdrawal.

Abrupt withdrawal, after high doses or long use, can result in an acute brain syndrome with disorientation and delirium, a paranoid psychosis and sometimes convulsions. Rapid withdrawal from low-dose treatment causes insomnia, anxiety, tremor and sweating, symptoms similar to those for which the benzodiazepine may have been first prescribed. Additional symptoms include nausea, heightened sensitivity to light and sound, sense of imbalance as on a rocking boat, which may impair mobility, peculiar and frightening sensory illusions, tinnitus, paraesthesia, depersonalisation and derealisation. These can last for weeks and full recovery may take one to two years after long-term treatment. Here a careful plan of slow and phased withdrawal, using diazepam at an equivalent dose (for instance 10 mg diazepam to 1 mg lorazepam), with concurrent support in a self-help group and relaxation classes is helpful. Start by reducing the dose by one-tenth every two weeks in out-patients or every week in in-patients. Some will feel better as the dose is reduced, but be prepared to reduce more slowly in those who suffer withdrawal symptoms.

Benzodiazepines are not harmless sedatives and hypnotics. They should be prescribed for a defined purpose within a plan of management. Prescribe for a finite period, for example two weeks, and then review their effects and only renew the prescription with justification. If treatment continues after dependence has begun to develop, the initial therapeutic effects become at least partly lost, and as each dose wears off the patient may experience a rebound exacerbation of the pre-existing condition to a more severe level than ever. Attacks of panic may occur whenever a short-acting drug such as lorazepam is wearing off. But at the same time it must be remembered that not every patient becomes dependent and, of those who do, not all take ever-increasing doses. Work with two or three from the large range of these drugs available and get to know a short-acting and a long-acting type.

Benzodiazepines are closely related compounds, all with the same ring structure (Fig. 8) to which atoms or radicals like -H, -OH, -CH$_3$, -Cl are attached at different points (see Table 2). In metabolism -CH$_3$ radicals can be removed (demethylation) and the active drug is turned into another active substance. Diazepam, medazepam, chlordiazepoxide

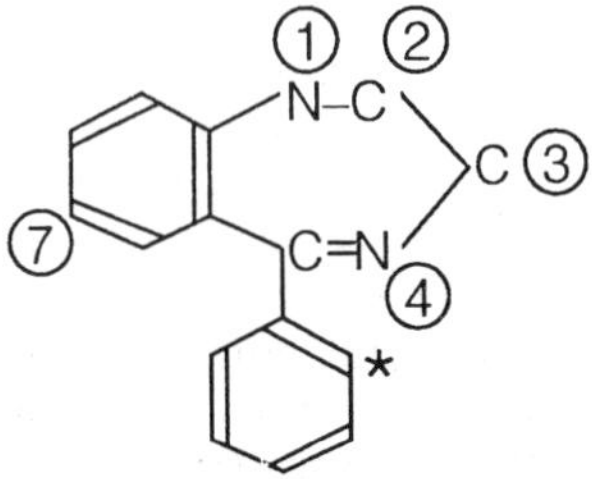

Fig. 8   The benzodiazepine structure

TABLE 2
Variations in benzodiazepine ground plan

Drug	Position (see Fig. 8)					
	1	2	3	4	7	*
Chlordiazepoxide	-	$NH.CH_3$	H_2	O	Cl	-
Diazepam	CH_3	O	H_2	-	Cl	-
Medazepam	CH_3	H_2	H_2	-	Cl	-
Temazepam	CH_3	O	OH	-	Cl	-
Oxazepam	H	O	H.OH	-	Cl	-
Lorazepam	H	O	H.OH	-	Cl	Cl
Clonazepam	H	O	H_2	-	NO_2	Cl
Nitrazepam	H	O	H_2	-	NO_2	-
Flurazepam	$(CH_2)_2N(C_2H_5)_2$	O	H_2	-	Cl	F
Clorazepate	H	OH.OK	H.COOK	-	Cl	-
Triazolam	triazolo	-	-	Cl	Cl	-

Note: the first three structures give rise to oxazepam; lorazepam is chloro-oxazepam, as clonazepam is chloronitrazepam.

and clorazepate all give rise to N-desmethyldiazepam (nordiazepam), and this metabolite itself will accumulate having a half-life of several days. Benzodiazepines differ among themselves chiefly in potency, and in speed of inactivation and excretion. Temazepam for example is quickly converted to inactive glucuronide and excreted by the kidney and is therefore short-acting, and useful as a hypnotic. But diazepam is converted to nordiazepam, which is active and only slowly converted on to other substances which are inert and lost.

Difficulty in getting off to sleep can be treated with a rapid onset, short-acting benzodiazepine such as temazepam. After a good night's sedation the patient should wake fresh without hangover, drowsiness or dysphoria.

Unfortunately, some of the short-acting drugs can produce a withdrawal syndrome as they wear off, with confusion, depression or even psychotic symptoms. There was concern about this occurring with large doses of triazolam and the drug is no longer available for use in Britain.

Large doses of short-acting benzodiazepines cause tolerance in 3–14 days. On stopping treatment, two or three nights of insomnia will occur before natural sleep rhythm returns, and patients should be told this otherwise they will ask for more drug. Be wary of using longer-acting benzodiazepines as night sedation, because the drugs accumulate and have effects the next day. Benzodiazepines are for short-term control of insomnia.

Episodes of acute anxiety can be prevented with a single dose of diazepam which has both a rapid and a slow component of action. The patient must know the situations likely to provoke anxiety, and should practise once or twice before they take place, to get the dose and timing right. For example, 2 mg or 5 mg of diazepam by mouth taken one hour before a stressful situation might be helpful.

Persistent anxiety can be controlled or made tolerable with a regular low dose of a longer-acting benzodiazepine such as oxazepam or diazepam. Although lower doses produce tolerance less quickly than larger, dependence is still a risk and treatment should not be longer than four weeks. Since chronic anxiety usually fluctuates a good deal in severity, intermittent use of these drugs, which is preferable to regular use, is a practical course.

Benzodiazepines are not antidepressants and long-term use may increase the risk of depression. It is therefore important to determine whether the patient's anxiety is one aspect of a depressive illness, and if so to avoid benzodiazepines.

Anxiety is common in situations requiring adjustment such as after a bereavement. Here the use of a benzodiazepine may impair the person's ability to grieve or make the necessary adjustment, and the drugs should be avoided.

Benzodiazepines cause impairment of mental ability, amnesia, decreased psychomotor reactions and coordination, and, in the elderly, ataxia. In some personalities they result in disinhibition and even aggression. Avoid prescribing for personalities prone to dependency. Cimetidine blocks benzodiazepine oxidation in the liver and so potentiates the effects. Renal and liver disease increase sensitivity.

Alcohol interacts with benzodiazepines centrally, and they potentiate one another, with increased incoordination, disinhibition and aggression. Benzodiazepines cause respiratory depression, particularly in the elderly, and those with emphysema and bronchitis are made worse by them. Benzodiazepines still have a part to play in controlling human distress. Occasionally there will be circumstances where the evils of drug dependence are less than the disabling and painful symptoms of a psychiatric condition which cannot otherwise be ameliorated. A benzodiazepine may be better than alcohol, if that is the alternative for the patient. Patients should always be warned of the risks of dependence, the impairment of coordination, and the interactions with alcohol, and advised not to drink.

Diazepam is discussed in detail as the type drug.

Diazepam

Diazepam ('Diazemuls', 'Stesolid', 'Valium') may be used for:

- (a) alleviation of anxiety
- (b) treatment of insomnia associated with anxiety
- (c) relief of delirium tremens
- (d) relief of lysergic acid diethylamide (LSD) reactions
- (e) abreaction
- (f) control of status epilepticus.

A single oral dose of 5 or 10 mg, occasionally more, will dampen anxiety in half to one hour, or may be taken before an anxiety-provoking situation. This quick effect will wear off in about four hours. The drug is metabolised to a less potent but more persistent anxiolytic. Repeated doses of 2 mg or more can be given on a regular schedule, twice or three times daily, when the main benefit will come from the accumulation of the less potent metabolite, which builds over the course of two weeks and is slow to disappear when treatment is stopped. Prescribe the smallest dose that will relieve symptoms. Avoid giving more than 30 mg per day and review the dosage weekly.

Diazepam can be used for insomnia, particularly when the problem is getting off to sleep, but its metabolites may produce hangover effects next morning, especially when used on successive nights. Temazepam is better. Assess critically whether patients taking regular daytime diazepam need separate night sedation or, likewise, whether patients taking regular night sedation need daytime sedation. In acute stress, or to induce relaxation in a behavioural desensitisation programme, or in abreaction, 10 mg or even 20 mg can be given intramuscularly or intravenously.

For delirium tremens and for reactions to LSD, 10 mg parenterally is repeated until control is achieved, and then oral doses used to maintain control until the acute state has remitted.

Diazepam is the treatment of choice for status epilepticus (see p. 159), by slow intravenous infusion or, in infants, by rectal infusion. Other benzodiazepines are not used in this way or in delirium tremens, but clonazepam can be a useful drug for epilepsy.

Side-effects and interactions

Tiredness or sleepiness may develop after some days, particularly on higher doses, or a morning hangover feeling. Ataxia and dizziness are less common. Pain in the legs has been noted in some elderly patients. Nausea and headache have been reported in others. In a few patients irritability or aggressive behaviour appears. Benzodiazepines should be avoided in those with a history of personality disorder or drug or alcohol abuse. In some, anxiety may even be increased. Drug dependence develops on higher doses and withdrawal symptoms appear a week or so after the drug is stopped. Sudden withdrawal may provoke fits.

Diazepam is less suitable for the elderly because of the greater risk of mental confusion, ataxia or falls, or in the presence of cardio-respiratory disorders as respiration is depressed.

Preparations

Tablets: 2 mg, 5 mg, 10 mg
Capsules: 2 mg, 5 mg
Elixir: 2 mg/5 ml
Injection: 5 mg/ml
Rectal solution: 2 mg/ml, 4 mg/ml

Other anxiolytics

*Alprazolam ('Xanax') –
  tablets: 0.25 mg, 0.5 mg (maximum daily dose 3 mg)
*Bromazepam ('Lexotan') –
  tablets: 1.5 mg, 3 mg (maximum daily dose 18 mg)
†Chlordiazepoxide ('Librium') –
  tablets: 5 mg, 10 mg, 25 mg (maximum daily dose 60 mg)
  capsules: 5 mg, 10 mg
*Clobazam ('Frisium') –
  capsules: 10 mg (maximum daily dose 30 mg)
*Clorazepate ('Tranxene') –
  capsules: 7.5 mg, 15 mg (maximum daily dose 22.5 mg)
*Ketazolam ('Anxon') –
  capsules: 15 mg, 30 mg (maximum daily dose 60 mg)
†Lorazepam ('Ativan') –
  tablets: 1 mg, 2.5 mg
  injection: 4 mg/ml (maximum daily dose 5 mg)
  withdrawal symptoms are common
*Medazepam ('Nobrium') –
  capsules: 5 mg, 10 mg (maximum daily dose 30 mg)
†Midazolam ('Hypnovel') –
  ampoules: 10 mg/2 ml, 10 mg/5 ml
†Oxazepam ('Oxanid') –
  tablets: 10 mg, 15 mg, 30 mg (maximum daily dose 90 mg)
  capsules: 30 mg

Note. The benzodiazepine brands marked with an asterisk are
not available at National Health Service expense. Drugs marked
with a dagger may only be prescribed under generic (not brand)
names.

Hypnotics

Short-acting

*Lormetazepam –
  tablets: 1 mg (maximum daily dose 1 mg)
†Temazepam ('Normison') –
  tablets: 10 mg, 20 mg (maximum daily dose 30 mg)
  capsules: 10 mg, 15 mg, 20 mg (maximum daily dose 30 mg)
  elixir: 10 mg/5 ml

Longer-acting

†Nitrazepam ('Mogadon') –
  tablets: 5 mg (maximum daily dose 10 mg)
  capsules: 5 mg
  suspension: 2.5 mg/5 ml
*Flunitrazepam ('Rohypnol') –
  tablets: 1 mg (maximum daily dose 1 mg)
*Flurazepam ('Dalmane') –
  capsules: 15 mg, 30 mg (maximum daily dose 30 mg)

Note. The benzodiazepine brands marked with an asterisk are not available at National Health Service expense. Drugs marked with a dagger may only be prescribed under generic (not brand) names.

Azaspirodecanediones

Buspirone

This is a new class of drugs which act primarily as partial agonists at 5-HT-1A receptors both pre- and post-synaptically. They reduce 5-HT function in the brain. They tend also to be antagonists at dopamine D-2 receptors.

Buspirone ('Buspar') is the first available drug in this class and has mild anti-anxiety effects which develop within one to two weeks of treatment. The recommended dose is 5–10 mg thrice daily. Claims are made for its uses as an adjunct to MARIs in depression and obsessive–compulsive disorder, but these remain to be proved. Tolerance and problematic withdrawal symptoms do not develop but the drug does not relieve benzodiazepine withdrawal symptoms. The side-effects include nausea, dizziness and headaches.

Preparations

Tablets: 5 mg, 10 mg

Cyclopyrrolones

Zopiclone

This group of compounds is structurally different from the benzodiazepines, but interacts with the same part of the GABA-A receptor, and has similar properties to the benzodiazepines.

Zopiclone ('Zimovane') is a sedative drug with a short half-life, suitable for night sedation. The dependence risk is not known but it should not be used for longer than four weeks. It should be used with the same precautions as the benzodiazepines and not prescribed to those with a history of substance abuse or personality disorder, or those who are still drinking alcohol. The side-effects include a bitter taste, nausea and vomiting. Irritability, depression, amnesia and hallucinations have also been reported. One or two tablets are prescribed at night.

Preparations

Tablets: 7.5 mg

Chloral hydrate ('Noctec', 'Welldorm')

Chloral hydrate is metabolised in the body to the chlorine-substituted alcohol, trichlorethanol. This is a safe hypnotic, with few side-effects, short-acting and without hangover, and is particularly suitable for the elderly and physically frail. Because of the risk of dependency it should be prescribed with the same caution as the benzodiazepines. Only use in the short term and avoid if there is severe cardiac, renal or hepatic disease.

Taken in water the mixture (0.5–2 g for insomnia) can be unpleasant to swallow because of the taste and causes gastric irritation. The addition of milk may help but a capsule ('Noctec') or tablet ('Welldorm') is better tolerated.

Preparations

Tablets: chloral betaine: 707 mg = 414 mg chloral hydrate
Capsules: 500 mg
Chloral mixture BPC: 0.5 g/5 ml
Elixir: 143 mg/5 ml
A related substance, triclofos sodium, is tasteless and causes less gastric irritation. The hypnotic dose is 1–2 g.
Tablets: 500 mg
Elixir: 500 mg/5 ml

Barbiturates

Barbiturates are used in psychiatry for anaesthesia for electroconvulsive therapy, to control epilepsy, sometimes for abreaction, and only rarely for symptom control, because they carry serious risks of drug dependence and toxicity in overdose.

The different members of the barbiturate group vary principally in the speed with which they are metabolised by the liver and excreted in the urine; the more slowly metabolised barbiturates are more likely to cause hangovers and to accumulate. Accumulation can cause a chronic brain syndrome – drowsiness, disorientation, muddled thinking, slurred speech and ataxia. The elderly are especially liable because their bodies deal slowly with drugs.

When tolerance develops, the same dose no longer relieves the symptoms. The doctor then has to consider whether to increase the dose to achieve control of symptoms, bearing in mind the risk of dependence by step-wise increase of dose, or to stop barbiturates and use some other drug. In the dependent state the patient becomes irritable and moody whenever doses are not maintained. Cutting down the dose results in sleeplessness, agitation, complaints of tension, depression and even grand mal fits if the reduction is rapid. The drug must never be stopped abruptly, but the dose reduced slowly over about six weeks.

Amylobarbitone sodium ('Sodium Amytal')

This drug is now used only rarely (and when major tranquillisers have failed) to control severe emotional and behavioural disturbance and for short periods of a few days. Start with 400 mg or 600 mg orally and then 200 mg four-hourly. More rapid control is gained by a single intramuscular or slow intravenous dose of 250 mg or more (up to 0.5 g intramuscularly or 1 g intravenously), the dose being judged by its almost immediate effect and repeated in a revised dose when the effect begins to wear off. Combined barbiturate and major tranquilliser can prove dramatically effective when the latter alone achieves little.

Side-effects and interactions

Be cautious if renal or liver disease is present since these two organs normally terminate barbiturate action. Barbiturates are respiratory depressants and unsuitable in chronic bronchitis. Do not give to the elderly patient because of the risk of inducing disorientation.

Alcohol potentiates their effect and the two should never be taken together. The rare disease, porphyria, is exacerbated by them. Barbiturates stimulate liver enzymes and this leads to increased metabolism of other drugs. In the blood they may displace other drugs from their binding to plasma albumin.

The prescribing of barbiturates, as outlined above, is exceptional: always remember the risks of drug dependence, of death from accidental poisoning, especially in the elderly, the ill and the alcoholic, and the risk of suicide.

Preparations

Tablets: 60 mg, 200 mg
Capsules: 60 mg, 200 mg
Injection: 250 mg and 500 mg powder in ampoules (for reconstitution)

Paraldehyde

This is a rapidly acting hypnotic and anticonvulsant which is safe in the presence of poor renal function since it is excreted predominantly in the breath.

Its use in the control of excitement is now obsolete because it is so unpleasant, and injection of more than 5 ml at one site can cause local necrosis and abscess formation.

It can be used to control status epilepticus and delirium tremens; but it can induce dependence.

People dislike its smell and taste. A rectal infusion, given as a 10% enema and saline, avoids this but may cause local irritation. A similar reaction can occur when taken orally. If giving it by deep intramuscular injection, beware of using plastic syringes, which it dissolves, and of damage to the sciatic nerve; abscess formation is a particular risk. Whichever method, the dose is 5–10 ml (not more than 5 ml at one injection site). Avoid if liver damage or lung disease is present. The drug interacts with disulfiram (see p. 298).

Preparations

Paraldehyde draft BPC: 4 ml, 50 ml
Injection: 5 ml ampoule, 10 ml ampoule

Further reading

PRIEST, R. G. & MONTGOMERY, S. A. (1988)   Benzodiazepines and
    dependence: a college statement. *Psychiatric Bulletin,* **12**, 107–108.
RICKELS, K., SCHWEIZER, E., CASE, G., *et al* (1990) Long term therapeutic
    use of benzodiazepines. I: effects of abrupt discontinuation. *Archives
    of General Psychiatry,* **47**, 899–907.

28   Stimulants and appetite suppressants

The amphetamines are a group of compounds related to d-alpha-methyl-phenylethylamine (dexamphetamine) which share an action to release DA, NA or 5-HT from neuronal stores. The mechanism by which they do this is unclear, but they may reverse the normal reuptake mechanism. They differ in the extent to which they release NA, DA or 5-HT, and at higher doses some are also MAOIs and block the reuptake of the transmitters. Dexamphetamine, methyl-phenidate, and pemoline act mainly upon DA and to a lesser extent NA release. They are psychostimulants and reduce appetite. Cocaine has similar effects, as well as being a local anaesthetic. Fenfluramine acts mainly upon 5-HT release, is sedative and reduces food intake, increasing satiety.

The stimulant amphetamines are of great interest to psychiatry because in low doses they produce euphoria similar to hypomania, but with reduced appetite; higher doses can produce a condition resembling paranoid schizophrenia, together with stereotyped behaviour similar to catatonic symptoms. They are also drugs of abuse and dependence.

Dexamphetamine

Dexamphetamine ('Dexedrine') is used for:

(a)   narcolepsy
(b)   Kleine-Levin syndromes

(c)   hyperkinetic children
(d)   epilepsy, to increase alertness.

Amphetamines are used, often illegally, for their euphoriant action and for counteracting fatigue or for suppressing appetite. Tolerance for these effects, especially the euphoriant effect, develops rapidly. On withdrawal, lethargy and depression occur. There is therefore a serious risk of inducing dependence. For this reason, the prescription of amphetamine is controlled under Schedule 2 of the Misuse of Drugs Act. This stimulant should not be used to treat depression or as an appetite suppressant because of the risk of dependence, abuse and psychosis.

To treat narcolepsy or Kleine-Levin syndrome start with 10 mg in the morning and increase by 10 mg steps each week until control is achieved or a maximum of 50 mg per day reached. Clomipramine may be even more effective.

For children with hyperkinesis (see Chapter 15 – Disorders of childhood) start with 2.5 mg in the morning and increase by weekly steps of 2.5 mg to a maximum of 20 mg daily, divided into two or three doses daily.

Dexamphetamine (5 mg two or three times a day) can reverse the drowsiness and inattention caused by anticonvulsant drugs.

The drug may cause insomnia, especially if taken late in the day. Misery and tearfulness can appear, usually transiently, in children taking therapeutic doses.

Long-term use in high dosage may retard children's growth because of appetite suppression. Height and weight must therefore be measured regularly.

High doses can cause perseveration of attention with consequent learning problems, so concentration must be monitored. Tics and stereotyped behaviour can be made worse. Agitation, excitement and even a paranoid psychosis with hallucinations occur in adults. Tachycardia, palpitations and a rise in blood pressure can all occur, so heart rate and blood pressure need to be examined regularly.

Beware of increasing tolerance and the development of psychological dependence. A depressive mood swing on stopping can occur. Beware of parents abusing a child by giving excessive doses.

The drug should not be given to people with a history of cardiovascular disease, hypertension, tics or drug dependence. It causes hypertensive and hyperpyrexial reactions if given with an MAOI. Amphetamine antagonises the antihypertensive effect of guanethidine.

Preparations

Tablets: 5 mg

Pemoline

Pemoline ('Volital') is a stimulant, like dexamphetamine but rather less potent, and is used in children who are hyperkinetic or epileptic, to increase alertness. Pemoline is longer-acting so that once-daily dosage is enough: 0.5 to 2.0 mg/kg (usually 20–80 mg daily) for children of 6–15 years. Begin with 20 mg daily and increase by 20 mg weekly, until the best response is achieved.

It is not controlled under the Misuse of Drugs Act.

Preparations

Tablets: 20 mg

Appetite suppressants

Most drugs marketed to assist in the treatment of obesity are stimulants such as diethylpropion ('Tenuate') and phentermine ('Duromine') and should not be prescribed. Fenfluramine, however, is sedative and carries much less risk of inducing dependence or psychosis. It is available as either the racemic mixture dl-fenfluramine or as dexfenfluramine.

dl-Fenfluramine

dl-Fenfluramine ('Ponderax') is prescribed as sustained-release capsules in a dose of 60 mg daily, raised to 120 mg and then to 180 mg at two-week intervals, if necessary. Treatment must stop at 12 weeks, with stepwise reduction every few days.

Tiredness, sedation, diarrhoea, dizziness and headache are the most likely side-effects, and tolerance is possible. It can potentiate drugs used in the treatment of hypertension and also interacts with MAOIs with the risk of excitement, hypertension and hyperpyrexia. It is therefore best avoided when other medical treatments are necessary.

Depression may occur after abrupt cessation, and mania has also been reported.

Preparations

Capsule (slow release): 60 mg dl-fenfluramine

Dexfenfluramine

Dexfenfluramine ('Adifax') is the dextro isomer active for the release of 5-HT. It is thus twice as potent as the dl-form for reducing appetite. The dose is 15 mg, twice daily. This should not be continued beyond three months. However, some authorities view this restriction as unnecessary because of the low risk of abuse. The drug has been used in patients who became obese on antipsychotic drugs; weight loss occurred without deterioration of the mental state.

The side-effects are dry mouth, nausea, and diarrhoea. Drowsiness, headache and dizziness also occur. Depression may occur with abrupt cessation. Other interactions occur as with the dl-mixture, although psychotic reactions are less likely. Reversible pulmonary hypertension may occur rarely.

Preparations

Dexfenfluramine –
    tablets: 15 mg

Caffeine

Caffeine has stimulant but not euphoriant properties. It increases arousal and is an ingredient of certain compound tablets that would otherwise be sedative, for instance painkillers. Its alerting properties are thought to be due to its action as an antagonist of adenosine at receptors in the brain. It also inhibits phosphodiesterase, causing increased levels of c-AMP, but this action appears at higher concentrations.

Caffeine has a half-life of about five hours. Hence if consumed in the evening it can disturb sleep throughout the night; this effect is more noticeable with increasing age.

Further reading

CHIARELLO, R. J. & COLE, J. O. (1987) The use of psychostimulants in general psychiatry. *Archives of General Psychiatry*, **44**, 286–295.

29 Anticonvulsants

'Anticonvulsants' is the term given to a diverse group of chemicals which can control fits. The mechanisms of their anticonvulsant actions, preventing the spread of abnormal excitation in the brain, are not all known. Some may stabilise neuronal excitability by blocking the exchange of ions across membranes, some by altering neurotransmitter levels. Barbiturates and phenytoin are thought to have an effect on membranes. Benzodiazepines, valproate, barbiturates, and vigabatrin are believed to enhance GABA mechanisms, lamotrigine to reduce the excitatory transmitter glutamate.

Anticonvulsants are small, liquid-soluble molecules absorbed from the gut with ease. They differ from each other in their rates of renal excretion, hepatic metabolism and fat solubility, factors determining drug levels in blood and brain. Carbamazepine and sodium valproate for example are rapidly metabolised and should be taken several times a day to maintain a therapeutic blood level, although brain drug levels may not fluctuate as rapidly as serum levels. In contrast phenytoin, phenobarbitone and primidone are slowly metabolised and can be taken in a single, daily dose. Some days are needed after a change of dose to reach a new equilibrium. This is a reason why improvement may be delayed a week or so after increasing a dose.

Competitive inhibition can result in one drug causing a rise in the serum level of another while enzyme induction can cause a decrease. Phenytoin, barbiturates and carbamazepine in particular have these properties.

Most anticonvulsant drugs circulate in the blood partly free and partly bound to plasma proteins, the ratio of free to bound drug being a constant. When only one drug is taken, measuring the total serum concentration will serve as an estimate of free drug, the pharmacologically active fraction. But when more than one drug is taken, binding sites on the plasma protein may be competed for and one drug may displace another. Carbamazepine may displace phenytoin for instance. This results in a higher fraction of the total serum phenytoin being unbound and active with the possibility of toxicity from a dose formerly safe.

Metabolic adjustments including enzyme changes may take weeks to reach a steady state so clinical changes must be judged over a lengthy period.

Some drug-induced metabolic changes can result in new disease. A few anticonvulsants stimulate the production of liver enzymes which increases the metabolism of calciferol and prevents the conversion of dietary vitamin D to the metabolically active chemical. A person with a poor vitamin intake and no sunshine may be tipped into vitamin deficiency by long-term phenytoin or phenobarbitone. Phenytoin may divert folate from its metabolic role resulting in a macrocytic anaemia. Porphyria may be precipitated by phenobarbitone, carbamazepine or phenytoin. Blood dyscrasias occur occasionally with nearly all the anticonvulsants.

In the past, grand mal and partial seizures were usually well controlled by barbiturates or phenytoin. Phenytoin, despite its side-effects, was preferred because of phenobarbitone's effects of sedation, increased irritability and cognitive impairment. Nowadays, both carbamazepine and sodium valproate are probably better because of fewer side-effects. Petit mal responds to ethosuximide or sodium valproate. Temporal lobe epilepsy is more difficult to control; a combination of two drugs may be unavoidable.

Aim to use one drug to control fits (see Table 3). Add a second only when one drug by itself has failed after a systematic trial. The prescription of more than two drugs concurrently results in a high frequency of side-effects, drug interactions, poor compliance and muddle about which drug is causing what effect.

TABLE 3
Guidelines for choice of drugs

Seizure type	First choice	Second choice
Grand mal (primary generalised)	Carbamazepine Phenytoin Sodium valproate	Phenobarbitone Primidone
Petit mal	Ethosuximide Sodium valproate	Clonazepam
Partial (focal) motor/sensory	Carbamazepine Phenytoin Sodium valproate	Phenobarbitone Primidone
Temporal lobe (partial complex)	Carbamazepine Phenytoin	Phenobarbitone Primidone
Myoclonic/atonic	Sodium valproate Clonazepam	Ethosuximide
Status epilepticus	Diazepam	(Chlormethiazole Paraldehyde)

Carbamazepine

Carbamazepine ('Tegretol') may be used for:

    (a)   all forms of epilepsy excepting petit mal
    (b)   mood disturbance (see p. 90)
    (c)   trigeminal neuralgia.

For adults, give 200 mg daily, increasing the dose by 200 mg every two or three days, depending on response. For most people 800–1200 mg is adequate but a few may require 1600 mg a day.

    For children the dose ranges between 100 mg for infants to 1000 mg for 15-year-olds. Aim for a plasma level of 4–12 mg/l, but be more guided by clinical response and tolerance of side-effects. Carbamazepine induces its own catabolic enzymes so serum levels may decline after a time on a constant dose with the possibility of fits recurring. Carbamazepine should be avoided with atrio-ventricular conduction disorders and porphyrias.

Side-effects and interactions

Gastrointestinal disturbances, nausea, headache, dizziness, drowsiness, ataxia, confusion, nystagmus, diplopia and fluid retention. Hyponatraemia occurs occasionally. A reduction in white cell count is common but blood dyscrasias with agranulocytosis can occur. A weekly blood count for the first month of treatment is advised. Patients should report signs of infection, a sore throat or rash, which should prompt a full blood count. An itchy erythematous rash develops in about 5% and the drug should be stopped because of the rare possibility of Stevens-Johnson syndrome. Expert advice should be sought.

It is related to imipramine and may improve mood. Because of this similarity, it should not be given with an MAOI. Carbamazepine induces liver enzymes, thereby reducing levels of clonazepam, ethosuximide and sodium valproate if taken concurrently with them. In the same way carbamazepine lessens the effectiveness of other drugs including psychotropic drugs, and itself. The dose of oral contraceptives and of warfarin may need raising. Some drugs, for example cimetidine, inhibit the metabolism of carbamazepine, so increasing the serum level. Because of the risk of neural-tube defects it should be avoided in pregnancy.

Preparations

Tablets: 100 mg, 200 mg, 400 mg
Chewable tablets: 100 mg, 200 mg
Slow-release tablets: 200 mg, 400 mg
Liquid: 100 mg per 5 ml

Phenytoin

Phenytoin ('Epanutin') may be used for all types of epilepsy except petit mal.

For adults, and children over six years, 100 mg daily in one or two doses may be increased gradually to 600 mg daily, depending on response. For children under six years, 5–8 mg/kg daily in one or two doses is recommended.

Several weeks are required to reach a stable level after each dose increase because of the long half-life. Phenytoin has a narrow therapeutic index. A small increase in dose may produce a large and toxic increase in serum level and increase of dose should be linked with plasma monitoring. Because of saturation of the liver enzymes, aim for plasma levels of 10–20 mg/l (40–80 micromol/l). Patients sensitive to their facial appearance, adolescents especially, may not tolerate the facial coarsening, gum hyperplasia, acne and hirsutism.

Side-effects and interactions

Gastric upsets are common. At higher doses nystagmus, diplopia, vertigo, ataxic gait, and other cerebellar signs may occur; also an acute brain syndrome, sometimes accompanied by dystonia and choreo-athetosis. Hyperplasia of gums develops in 20% of those on chronic treatment. Hirsutism, peripheral neuritis, skin rash and rarely folate deficiency anaemia may develop. The folate deficiency can be treated with folic acid, permitting continuation of phenytoin.

Avoid giving during pregnancy; primidone is preferable. Carbamazepine levels are lowered by concurrent prescription of phenytoin. Phenobarbitone interaction is complex, so in combined treatment check both drug levels after the dose of one is changed. Avoid rapid withdrawal.

Preparations

Tablets: 50 mg, 100 mg
Capsules: 25 mg, 50 mg, 100 mg, 300 mg
Chewable tablets (paediatric): 50 mg
Suspension: 30 mg per 5 ml
Injection: 50 mg per ml in 5 ml ampoule (irritant to tissues)

Sodium valproate

Sodium valproate ('Epilim') may be used for all forms of epilepsy. For adults give 200 mg three times a day, increasing by 200 mg every third day according to response. Control of fits usually appears at 800–1400 mg, but severe cases may need up to 2500 mg daily. For children the dose range is 400–1200 mg, and for infants up to three years, 20–30 mg/kg per day. Clinical response is the best guide to dose. There is much individual variation and no clear therapeutic range. Serum levels are useful for identifying the poor complier and for deciding to change to another drug when fit control is not achieved with a serum level above 150 mg/l.

Side-effects and interactions

Drowsiness, nausea, vomiting, increase in appetite and weight gain. Fatal cases of acute liver disease have been reported, usually in patients with severe epilepsy who were or had been taking other anticonvulsants in combination. If there is any history of liver disease, check liver function regularly; if liver disease is active, avoid altogether. Serum phenobarbitone levels are raised when valproate is given with primidone or phenobarbitone, intensifying sedation. Sedation is marked when benzodiazepines are combined with valproate. It should be avoided in pregnancy because of the risk of neural-tube defect.

Preparations

Tablets: 100 mg, 200 mg, 500 mg
Syrup and liquid: 200 mg per 6 ml
Injection: 400 mg per vial to mix with 4 ml water in ampoule

Phenobarbitone

Phenobarbitone may be used for all forms of epilepsy, except petit mal. Phenobarbitone has now been superseded by phenytoin and carbamazepine as the drug of first choice in grand mal and partial seizures.

Where it is to be used, the adult dose is 60–200 mg a day, and for children 5–8 mg/kg body weight given at night to avoid sedation. Aim for a plasma level of 15–40 mg/l (60–180 micromol/l). The drug is slowly metabolised by liver hydroxylases and takes several days to reach a stable blood level.

Side-effects and interactions

The initial sedation lessens as tolerance develops. Rarely, dexamphetamine is given to lessen sedation. Nystagmus, ataxia and confusion may develop with big doses, especially in the elderly. Adults may show personality changes and children become irritable and overactive. Megaloblastic anaemia has been reported.

Oversedation may occur in the elderly and infirm. Breast-fed babies can become sleepy. Unsuitable for alcoholics and those with impaired liver function. Phenobarbitone may reduce levels of other drugs by inducing liver hydroxylase. However, it may decrease the inactivation of phenytoin and raise its serum level.

Preparations

Tablets: 15 mg, 30 mg, 60 mg, 100 mg
Elixir: 15 mg per 5 ml
Injection (phenobarbitone sodium, gardenal sodium):
  200 mg per 1 ml ampoule (must be diluted before
  intravenous use)

Primidone

Primidone ('Mysoline') is converted to phenobarbitone in
the liver, and this is why it is an anticonvulsant. Therefore
do not combine it with phenobarbitone in treatment: note
that all its side-effects are the same but more pronounced.
It can be used for all forms of epilepsy except petit mal.
Start with low doses, given at night to minimise side-effects:
for adults 125 mg increasing every third day by 125 mg to
a level of 500–1500 mg daily; and for children allow
5–20 mg/kg body weight.

Preparations

Tablets: 250 mg
Oral suspension: 250 mg per 5 ml

Ethosuximide

Ethosuximide ('Emeside', 'Zarontin') is mainly used for
petit mal but may be tried in myoclonic and other seizures.
For adults start with 500 mg daily, increasing by 500 mg
each week to 2000 mg according to response. In children
under six years begin with 250 mg daily, increasing to
1000 mg. Aim for a plasma level of 40–120 mg/l (300–700
micromol/l). Complete suppression of fits occurs in 50%
of cases and partial in 25%. If other types of fit co-exist,
combine with carbamazepine, phenytoin or primidone.

Side-effects and interactions

Nausea, anorexia, headache, apathy, dizziness, sleepiness, mood changes, which are usually mild and diminish, skin rashes, and blood disorders may all occur. Carbamazepine decreases plasma concentrations of ethosuximide, and sodium valproate increases them.

Preparations

Capsules: 250 mg
Syrup: 250 mg per 5 ml

Clonazepam

Clonazepam ('Rivotril') can be used for all forms of epilepsy. Clonazepam is a benzodiazepine with a long half-life. For adults start with 0.5 mg daily, increasing by 0.5 mg every three days to a daily dose of 4–8 mg, depending on response. For children aged 5–12 years use 3–6 mg daily, for children aged 1–5 years, 1–3 mg daily. For status epilepticus, 1 mg by slow injection in an adult and 0.5 mg in a child is appropriate.

Side-effects and interactions

Drowsiness, which may be marked, can be lessened by giving at night and increasing the dose gradually. Giddiness, irritability, aggressiveness and diplopia are common.

Carbamazepine, phenobarbitone and phenytoin increase metabolism of clonazepam, and serum levels of clonazepam are lowered. Avoid rapid withdrawal, which can precipitate status epilepticus.

Preparations

Tablets: 0.5 mg, 2 mg
Injection: 1 mg per 1 ml ampoule (requires dilution)

Diazepam

Diazepam ('Valium', 'Diazemuls', 'Stesolid') may be used for status epilepticus. By intravenous infusion as a 0.5% solution at a rate of 2.5 mg (0.5 ml) each 30 seconds, a dose of 10–20 mg should be administered, depending on response. This may be repeated after 30–60 minutes and to maximum of 3 mg/kg over 24 hours. By rectum in solution, adults and children over three years, the dose is 10 mg. For children 1–3 years, 5 mg is recommended, repeated if necessary.

Side-effects

Mechanical ventilation may be required when given intravenously because of respiratory depression.

Preparations

Injection: 5 mg/ml in 2 ml ampoule
Injection (emulsion): 5 mg/ml in 2 ml ampoule ('Diazemuls')
Enema: 2 mg/ml and 4 mg/ml in 2.5 ml rectal tubes ('Stesolid')
(If diazepam or clonazepam is ineffectual in treating status epilepticus, chlormethiazole administered intravenously may be tried, or paraldehyde given intramuscularly or rectally (see p. 280).)

Lamotrigine

Use lamotrigine ('Lamictal') where partial or generalised tonic–clonic fits are poorly controlled by usual drugs and give concurrently. Said to act by stabilising neuronal membranes and inhibiting release of glutamate. Start with 50 mg, twice daily, for two weeks and then gradually increase to 200–400 mg daily. If given with sodium valproate, halve these doses.

Side-effects

Rashes (10%), diplopia, drowsiness, headache, gastro-intestinal upset and aggression may occur. Avoid in pregnancy and in hepatic and renal disease.

Preparations

Tablet: 50 mg, 100 mg

Vigabatrin

Vigabatrin ('Sabril') is recommended as an anticonvulsant for trial where other anti-epileptic drugs have failed. Give alone or in addition to current medication. It is thought to act by raising GABA in the central nervous system by inhibiting GABA transaminase. Give 1.5–4 g per day in single or twice daily doses.

Side-effects

Dizziness, unsteadiness, drowsiness and aggression may occur. Avoid in pregnancy, renal disease and in those with history of psychoses.

Preparations

Tablets: 500 mg

30 Drugs for substance misuse

Disulfiram

Disulfiram ('Antabuse') inhibits enzymes including aldehyde dehydrogenase. In combination with alcohol disulfiram produces head throbbing, palpitations, tachycardia, facial flush, nausea, vomiting and sometimes dyspnoea. This very unpleasant experience, due to accumulation of acetaldehyde, is the basis of its use to discourage drinking in the alcoholic Because of the potential severity of the reaction disulfiram is ideally restricted to the medically fit.

Disulfiram can be started with an alcohol challenge while medically supervised, or without. In present practice the challenge is usually dispensed with, and disulfiram 200 mg is taken each morning as an out-patient, the patient being informed of the reaction to expect when alcohol is drunk. If the reaction with alcohol is absent or modest when the patient has a drink the dose can be increased to 400 mg. Success depends on a motivated, compliant patient using disulfiram as one, but not the sole aid, to control. Compliance is improved by enlisting a family member to help.

The alternative approach, using a challenge, relies to some extent for its effectiveness on a strong aversive experience. Disulfiram is taken 800 mg on the first night, 600 mg on the second, 400 mg on the third, and thereafter 200 mg each day. On the fifth morning, one hour after the last dose, give 15 ml of 95% alcohol diluted with the patient's favourite alcoholic drink. Within two hours the unpleasant experience should occur. The aim is to make a deep impression. If there is no adverse reaction, the dose of disulfiram can be increased and the challenge repeated. After the successful challenge, continue disulfiram (200 mg, daily). The anti-alcohol effect lasts two days or more after the last dose of disulfiram. Severe reactions may be ended with 1 g ascorbic acid orally or intravenously, and an intravenous injection of an antihistamine such as mepyramine maleate (25 mg or 50 mg).

Side-effects and interactions

Drowsiness, fatigue, constipation, nausea, a garlic or metallic taste, smelly breath, loss of libido. A smaller dose may reduce side-effects. The drug can also cause depressive or hallucinatory symptoms, and rarely encephalopathy with confusion, neurological signs and abnormal electro-encephalogram. Such reactions are less common since the recommended dose was reduced to 200 mg daily. Disulfiram can exacerbate schizophrenia, perhaps because of its inhibition of the enzyme dopamine beta-hydroxylase which converts dopamine to noradrenaline. A severe alcohol reaction produces falling blood pressure, cardiac arrhythmias, collapse, and can be fatal. The small amounts of alcohol sometimes in oral medicines may produce a reaction and patients should be warned of this. A patient's card as for MAOI may be useful.

Disulfiram interferes with the metabolism of other drugs, notably barbiturates, diazepam, phenytoin, warfarin, pethidine, theophylline and metronidazole, increasing their pharmacological actions. Paraldehyde metabolism is blocked by disulfiram, yielding acetaldehyde, which produces a severe reaction. The interaction with tricyclic antidepressants increases their blood levels and also increases the effects of disulfiram.

Preparations

Tablets: 200 mg

Methadone

Methadone ('Physeptone'), a synthetic opiate, is employed in psychiatry to manage opiate addiction. It has a longer time course of action than heroin. Controlled withdrawal is then easier to achieve using an oral drug with less acute withdrawal symptoms.

The initial dose depends upon the level of previous drug use and dependence: 40 mg per day in divided doses is usually adequate to begin with. Most clinics do not find it necessary to prescribe more than 60 mg or 80 mg daily. The dose is then reduced at a rate negotiated with the patient with the aim of avoiding maintenance beyond six months. The prescriptions must comply with the controlled drugs regulations (see p. 180).

Side-effects and interactions

Methadone, with a longer period of action than morphine, has similar side-effects but is not as sedative.

It potentiates the sedative effects of alcohol, antidepressants, neuroleptics and other psychotropic drugs. Liver disease, renal disease, asthma and MAOI drugs are contraindications unless the reasons for long-term use are compelling. Hypertensive crises may occur with MAOI drugs.

Preparations

Tablets: 5 mg
Mixture: 1 mg/ml
Injection: 10 mg/ml ('Physeptone')

Clonidine

Clonidine ('Catapres'), a centrally acting alpha-2 adrenergic agonist used to treat hypertension and migraine, is a useful adjunct in opiate withdrawal, suppressing autonomic symptoms without producing euphoria. Practice varies widely in its use both in withdrawal in acute phase or in longer-term management. Methadone can be prescribed simultaneously. Dose 100–600 mcg daily.

When used in opiate detoxification (see p. 172), the blood pressure and pulse are monitored. Clonidine is commenced in a dose of 200 mcg orally. After one hour, a further 100 mcg is given and repeated to a maximum of 400 mcg in any four-hour period. Blood pressure is taken before each dose and the dose withheld if it is below 80/60.

Side-effects and interactions

The side-effects include hypotension, drowsiness, dry mouth, oedema, bradycardia and depression. Lactation may be inhibited. Peripheral vascular diseases may be worsened, for example in Reynaud's disease. Hypertensive crises may occur on rapid withdrawal. Some MARI antidepressants lessen its hypotensive effect.

Preparations

Tablets: 100 mcg, 300 mcg
Capsules (sustained release): 250 mcg

Lofexidine

Lofexidine is an alpha-2 adrenergic agonist which reduces anxiety, tremor and diarrhoea associated with opiate withdrawal. It may also lower pulse and blood pressure, though less than clonidine, and these must therefore be monitored. The starting dose is 0.2 mg repeated after one hour to a maximum of 0.4 mg four-hourly.

There may be a rebound increase in blood pressure on stopping lofexidine and the blood pressure should continue to be monitored.

Preparations

Tablets: 0.2 mg

Naltrexone

Naltrexone ('Nalorex') is an opiate receptor blocker, and therefore prevents the effects including the 'buzz' experienced after taking an opiate. It therefore removes the principal reason for taking opiates illicitly. It is used in the management of well-motivated and cooperative patients. It has two main uses in treating addiction. Firstly, it aids detoxification. By competing for opiate receptors it displaces methadone and other opiate drugs, and thereby produces acute withdrawal symptoms of full intensity which wane over the following three to five days.

Secondly, it may be used in long-term management of the drug-free patient after detoxification, the intention being to deter future use by antagonising the effects of opiate drugs that may be taken. Its use in this situation to prevent relapse has not been shown to be better than placebo.

Its use for detoxification should be as an in-patient with staff familiar with the treatment and after full explanation has been given to the patient (see p. 172). The patient should have already reduced their use of methadone to 30 mg daily or less. After observation for 24 hours without opiates the patient will show some withdrawal symptoms (see also p. 172). They are commenced on lofexidine or clonidine. Two hours later they receive naltrexone, 1 mg orally. This intensifies the withdrawal symptoms within 15 minutes and further lofexidine or clonidine is given. Two hours after the first dose of naltrexone, if well tolerated, a further 2 mg is given, and 2 hours later 5 mg naltrexone. Should the withdrawal symptoms become too distressing, either naltrexone is withheld or diazepam is given up to 20 mg orally four hourly. On day three clonidine or lofexidine is given followed one hour later by naltrexone 12.5 mg twice daily. On day four naltrexone 50 mg may be given, and lofexidine or clonidine used if necessary. Diazepam should not be necessary then.

Insomnia may remain a problem but hypnotics should be avoided if possible. Once on a full dose of 50 mg daily they may be discharged, to take 50 mg naltrexone daily for a further two weeks under out-patient supervision from specialist drugs workers. For long-term use naltrexone 50 mg daily is advised.

Side-effects and interactions

Nausea and vomiting, headache and sleeplessness may occur. Check hepatic function before and during long-term treatment and do not give if there is any impairment. Patients should carry a drug warning card in case they need opiates for genuine pain relief.

Preparations

Tablets: 50 mg

Chlormethiazole

Chlormethiazole ('Heminevrin') is a sedative drug. It is widely used to control delirium tremens and alcohol withdrawal symptoms, with close hospital supervision usually as an in-patient, but always with daily monitoring. The dosage should be adjusted so that the patient is sedated but rousable. It may start with 9–12 capsules on the first day administered as three or four separate doses. This is followed by 6–8 capsules the second day, 4–6 capsules the third day, and a gradual reduction in dosage until it is stopped altogether after a total of 7–9 days.

Side-effects

Addiction is the most serious problem and hence the drug should not be used for longer than nine days. Sneezing, nasal tingling or burning, and conjunctival irritation sometimes occur soon after starting treatment. These tend to improve with further doses and do not necessarily require cessation of treatment. Alcoholics who continue to drink when taking chlormethiazole risk fatal cardiorespiratory depression, therefore it should not be prescribed to alcoholics as out-patients except under daily supervision in a specialised clinic.

The drug is also used for short-term treatment of severe insomnia in the elderly in a dose of 1–2 capsules or 5–10 mls of syrup at night.

Preparations

Capsules: 192 mg chlormethiazole base (equivalent to 5 mg syrup)
Syrup: 250 mg/5 ml chlormethiazole edisylate
0.8% infusion: 8 mg/ml chlormethiazole edisylate

Further reading

CHARNEY, D. S., HENINGER, G. R. & KLEBER, H. D. (1986) The combined use of clonidine and naltrexone as a rapid, safe and effective form of abrupt withdrawal from methadone. *American Journal of Psychiatry*, **148**, 831–837.

GOSSOP, M. & STRANG, J. (1991) A comparison of the withdrawal responses of heroin and methadone addicts during detoxification. *British Journal of Psychiatry*, **158**, 697–699.

31 Beta-blockers

Beta adrenergic receptors are of three types: beta-1 in the heart; beta-2 in the bronchi, skeletal muscle and liver; and beta-3 in the adipose tissue. Some beta-blockers such as propranolol block all types. Others such as atenolol and metoprolol are relatively selective for beta-1 receptors, having less propensity to precipitate asthma than the others. The water-soluble drugs such as atenolol are less able to penetrate the brain and cause less sleep disturbance. Oxprenolol is a partial agonist and causes less slowing of the heart. The beneficial effects of beta-blockers in migraine are thought to be due to a separate action of blockade of 5-HT-1D receptors in cranial blood vessels.

Beta blockers are largely used in treating hypertension and cardiac arrythmias. They are also used to suppress somatic anxiety symptoms.

Propranolol

Propranolol ('Inderal', 'Apsolol', 'Berkolol') may be used for:

(a)   bodily symptoms of anxiety
(b)   fine tremor, as in anxiety, familial tremor
(c)   akathisia.

Propranalol acts by blocking peripheral beta-adrenergic receptors and in this way relieves rapid pulse, palpitations, sweating and tremor. Neurotic patients who are troubled mainly by the bodily symptoms of anxiety are therefore more likely to be helped by propranolol than those with mental symptoms of anxiety. Somatic symptoms arising from both acute panic attacks and chronic anxiety states can be relieved. The usual treatment is 10 mg, 20 mg or even 40 mg, three or four times daily by mouth, beginning with the lower dose. Even higher doses may be tolerated.

High doses of up to 1000 mg were claimed to be helpful in treating schizophrenia, but this is a drug interaction since propranolol interferes with the degradative metabolism of chlorpromazine, slowing the process.

Propranolol is effective in familial tremor and other tremors not caused by anxiety, including lithium-induced tremor. Interestingly, beta-2 agonists such as salbutamol and terbutaline may cause tremor and feelings of muscular tension. Propranolol, 20–40 mg daily, is used to treat drug-induced akathisia; the site of this action is thought to be central, since only the fat-soluble beta-blockers are effective, but the mechanism is unclear. Both specific B_1 and B_2 antagonists are effective. A B_1 antagonist such as metoprolol is preferable to reduce the risk of bronchospasm.

The beta-adrenergic blockade caused by propranolol reduces the pulse rate, but the rate should not go below 55 beats per minute. Bradycardia can be reversed by 1–2 mg of atropine intravenously. Treatment with propranolol should be discontinued by gradual dose reduction and not abrupt withdrawal, to avoid rebound tachycardia and hypertension.

Side-effects and contraindications

Propranolol causes few side-effects in the physically healthy person. Light-headedness, visual and tactile hallucinations, tinnitus, erythematous skin rash and purpura have been reported. Propranolol can precipitate heart failure. If there is a history of cardiac disease, a cardiologist's advice should be sought before prescribing propranolol for anxiety. The drug interferes with the recognition of hypoglycaemia in the diabetic by preventing sweating and tachycardia. It may cause tiredness, insomnia with nightmares and/or depressive symptoms, and coldness of the periphery.

Asthma and obstructive airways disease contraindicate its use because of the risk of acute bronchospasm.

Preparations

Tablets: 10 mg, 40 mg, 80 mg, 160 mg
Capsules (sustained release): 80 mg, 160 mg

Other related drugs

Atenolol ('Antipressan', 'Tenormin')

Tablets: 25 mg, 50 mg, 100 mg (100 mg maximum daily
  dose)

Oxprenolol ('Trasicor', 'Apsolox')

Tablets: 20 mg, 40 mg, 80 mg, 160 mg (160 mg maximum
  daily dose)
Capsules (sustained release): 160 mg

Further reading

DUMON, J-P., CATTEAU, J., LANVIN, F., *et al* (1992) Randomised, double-blind, crossover, placebo controlled comparison of propranolol and betaxolol in the treatment of neuroleptic-induced akathisia. *American Journal of Psychiatry*, **149**, 647–650.

LADER, M. (1988) Beta adrenoceptor antagonism in neuropsychiatry: an update. *Journal of Clinical Psychiatry*, **49**, 213–223.

32   Anti-androgens

The male sex hormones are testosterone and dihydro-testosterone, which is produced in the target tissues by the action of the enzyme testosterone 5-alpha-reductase. The male hormones or androgens support the sex drive in men and in women, whose main source of androgens is the adrenal gland. Receptors for androgens are present in the central nervous system as well as in the genitalia, and are important from before birth – when testosterone is thought to masculinise the brain and internal genitalia, and dihydrotestosterone to masculinise the external genitalia.

In testosterone 5-alpha-reductase deficiency, dihydro-testosterone is not produced, and the external genitalia at birth appear female. At puberty such individuals undergo a striking virilisation, the most surprising part of which is that their gender identity and psychosexual orientation are those of heterosexual males, despite having been reared as females – the Imperato-McGinley syndrome.

Androgen secretion from the testes is controlled by luteinising hormone (LH). Secretion of LH from the pituitary is inhibited by progestogens. Drugs such as cyproterone and medroxy-progesterone act both to reduce testosterone levels and to block its receptors.

Cyproterone

Cyproterone acetate ('Androcur'), a powerful anti-androgen and progesterone-like compound, competitively blocks androgens at receptor sites, including those in the brain, and reduces secretion of LH and testosterone. The reason for using the drug to control hypersexuality and deviant behaviour in the male is the assumption that such behaviour depends on androgen levels. Clinical experience suggests the drug can be useful in helping the well-motivated male patient to control deviant sexual behaviour.

Cyproterone may improve paedophilia, exhibitionism, fetishism, other deviant behaviour, and excessive demand for sexual intercourse if these practices are related to high sexual drive. Because of this, younger men are more likely to respond than older men. A dose of 100 mg daily (range 50–200 mg) is recommended but assess patients every few days after each dose change. Drug treatment should be combined with psychological treatment directed to encouraging motivation to change and alter sexual preoccupations.

The use of cyproterone raises ethical and legal problems because of its intended effect to control an important part of behaviour. The doctor should verify that the patient is fully informed of the side-effects and the nature of treatment. The Mental Health Act 1983 excludes sexual deviation as a recognised form of mental disorder, so that compulsory treatment cannot be given for this alone. When used to treat sexual aspects of mental illness in detained patients, cyproterone can be used without consent, provided a second opinion under Section 58 gives approval, after three months of treatment for mental disorder.

Side-effects and interactions

Tiredness is the main unwanted side-effect and is transient but gynaecomastia, which may be irreversible, occurs in 20% of those given the drug. Reversible infertility is common, with increased numbers of abnormal spermatozoa. Whether abnormal offspring are born to fathers taking cyproterone is unknown but the patient should be warned. Cyproterone may cause liver damage and so should not be used for patients with liver disease, and liver function should be checked.

Preparations

Tablets: 50 mg

Benperidol

Benperidol ('Anquil') can be used in place of haloperidol in disturbed psychotic states, especially when associated with disinhibition and hypersexuality. It is also used in personality disorders with sexual deviation or abnormal sexual preoccupations but its effectiveness has not yet been established. Side-effects are as for butyrophenones and dosage varies from 0.25–1.5 mg daily in divided doses.

Preparations

Tablets: 0.25 mg

Oestrogen implants

Oestrogen implants reduce male sex drive but cause side-effects including feminisation. They are no longer used and would be restricted by Section 57 of the Mental Health Act; this requires both consent and a second opinion, from an approved doctor, for the implantation of hormones to reduce sexual drive.

Medroxy-progesterone acetate

Medroxy-progesterone acetate ('Depo-Provera') has also been used to reduce testosterone levels and treat a variety of male sexual offenders with a high sex drive. However, it is not licenced for this use.

Goserelin

Goserelin, a long-acting analogue of LH, reduces LH and testosterone levels for one month after a single injection. Its use is not restricted by Section 57 of the Mental Health Act. It is judged not to be a hormone, and a distinction is made between injections and implantation, according to a court ruling.

Further reading

COOPER, A. J. (1986) Progestogens in the treatment of male sexual offenders: a review. *Canadian Journal of Psychiatry*, **31**, 73–79.

DYER, C. (1988) Mental Health Commission defeated over paedophile. *British Medical Journal*, **296**, 1660–1661.

GAGNE, P. (1981) Treatment of sex offenders with medroxy-progesterone acetate. *American Journal of Psychiatry*, **138**, 644–646.

IMPERATO-MCGINLEY, J., PETERSON, R. E., GAUTIER, T., *et al* (1979) Androgens and the evolution of male-gender identity among male pseudo-hermaphrodites with 5-alpha-reductase deficiency. *New England Journal of Medicine*, **300**, 1233–1237.

33 Vitamins

Prescribing vitamins for psychiatric patients is justified only when a vitamin deficiency state exists or there is strong suspicion that it does so. Vitamin deficiency states are uncommon in psychiatric patients but a diet of poor quality or quantity, over a lengthy period, can lead to deficiency in the B group, vitamin C, vitamin B_{12} and folic acid.

Such a state results from the unsupervised self-neglect which occurs with dementia, the elderly mentally ill, chronic schizophrenia, and long-standing alcoholism, or from the deliberate self-starvation of anorexia nervosa and the extreme dietary practices resulting from delusional beliefs. An adequate diet, if the patient will have it, and vitamin supplements are all that are required to manage the deficiency in the short-term. A multiple vitamin preparation containing ascorbic acid, nicotinamide, pyridoxine, riboflavine and thiamine is often used. Folic acid may have to be prescribed if anaemia is present and this needs to be confirmed by a low red cell folate. Plasma folate levels indicate only current intake, not past deficiency. Dietary stores of vitamin B_{12} are usually large enough to withstand several years of poor diet. Excessive intake of a vitamin may result from a delusion and be harmful and occasionally life-threatening, for example, excessive amounts of carrot juice causing vitamin A poisoning.

Some psychiatric conditions result from vitamin deficiencies, although this is rare in Britain. Alcoholism and a poor diet may cause a thiamine deficiency which, if not urgently treated, damages mid-brain structures resulting in Wernicke's encephalopathy and subsequent Korsakoff's syndrome. Thiamine, given with other vitamins, prevents the syndrome from developing and probably shortens the delirium. Treatment is an urgent matter.

Pellagra, with its psychosis and dementia, is a rare consequence of nicotinamide deficiency. Dementia and cognitive impairment associated with vitamin B_{12} and folic acid deficiency may respond partially to replacement therapy. The vitamin deficiency may not be causal but may result from a poor diet brought about by a dementia. Folate deficiency does lead to depression and irritability.

Pyridoxine is prescribed as a supplement to tryptophan, when used as an antidepressant, and also for pre-menstrual tension. But in neither case has its value been proved.

Many oral vitamin preparations are available. An injectable form, 'Parentrovite' is described here.

Parentrovite

Parentrovite may be used for:

(a) delirium tremens
(b) Wernicke's encephalopathy and Korsakoff's syndrome
(c) dietary deficiency states.

Parentrovite is a proprietary preparation of thiamine (B_1), riboflavine (B_2), pyridoxine (B_6), nicotinamide, and ascorbic acid (C) for parenteral use when vitamins are urgently required. For delirium tremens give pairs of intramuscular high-potency ampoules daily for five to seven days. Wernicke's encephalopathy as a medical emergency (see p. 132) requires a more vigorous approach with two to four pairs of ampoules every four to eight hours for up to 48 hours, depending on clinical response, followed by one pair of intravenous or intramuscular ampoules a day for five to seven days. For the less serious case and Korsakoff's psychosis, a pair of intramuscular high-potency ampoules once or twice daily for up to seven days is sufficient until oral vitamin treatment can be given. Use only intravenous preparations for intravenous use and intramuscular preparations for intramuscular use.

Side-effects and interactions

Parentrovite is safe to use. Facial flushing occasionally results. Very large amounts may cause mental excitement which subsides when treatment stops. Anaphylaxis has been reported. Pyridoxine may destabilise the L-dopa treatment of Parkinson's disease.

Preparations

Intravenous, high potency

Ampoule 1, 5 ml: thiamine 250 mg, riboflavine 4 mg, pyridoxine 50 mg
Ampoule 2, 5 ml: nicotinamide 160 mg, ascorbic acid 500 mg, dextrose monohydrate 1000 mg.

Intramuscular, high potency

Vitamin composition as for intravenous, high potency, but without dextrose, and with benzyl alcohol 140 mg in two ampoules of 3.5 ml.

Intramuscular, maintenance

Ampoule 1, 2 ml: thiamine 100 mg, riboflavine 4 mg, pyridoxine 50 mg, benzyl alcohol 80 mg
Ampoule 2, 2 ml: nicotinamide 160 mg, ascorbic acid 500 mg.

Appendix 1. Consent to treatment

In general all patients have the right to have a proposed treatment explained to them and to decide whether to accept it or not. But psychiatric patients can pose three kinds of difficulty here.

(a) Some psychiatric patients may consent although they have not understood the explanation or what they are agreeing to. Perhaps they agree to please the doctor, or are giving way to what they feel is pressure or they regard the treatment as a punishment which they believe they fully deserve. This is not real consent; it is termed incompetent and is not acceptable.

(b) Others fail to give consent not because they necessarily disagree but because the very nature of their illness makes it impossible. They may be mute, or in catatonic stupor or suffer from a state of continuous indecision about everything, or entertain bodily delusions, or have a marked thought disorder which makes it very difficult to be sure what they mean when they speak.

(c) Some refuse in clear consciousness and after discussion. They do not believe they are ill or need treatment, and they may fear side-effects of drugs or the way they are given.

Yet it may truly be in the patient's best interests to have the proposed treatment, even a matter of death if they do not have it.

Without 'real' consent, or with refusal, treatment would be an assault and illegal. The Mental Health Act (MHA) 1983 provides a way forward, a procedure allowing treatment of the non-consenting patient by making safeguards for both patient and medical and nursing staff. The patient must be detained under a section of the MHA (which means that certain abnormalities in mental state and related behaviour are recognised by two separate doctors). An informal patient in hospital may have to be detained for this purpose. This needs recommendations by a doctor approved under section 12 of the MHA as having special knowledge of psychiatry, and of another doctor who is not on the hospital staff, most often the family doctor, who knows the patient and an application by an approved social worker or nearest relative. Section 2 of the MHA, lasting 28 days, or section 3 lasting six months are, thus, completed; both can be cancelled at any time before they expire. Mentally abnormal offenders detained through a court under sections 36, 37, 38 or transferred from prisons under sections 47 or 48 also satisfy the legal requirements.

After three months the patient is then assessed by the independent doctor for second opinions (SOAD) approved by the Mental Health Act Commission (MHAC), and agreement for treatment given or not.

This procedure with second opinions can take time, especially at weekends. In dire emergency, common law allows doctors to act for the patient on their own initiative alone, avoiding the MHA's procedure. For example, medication is given under common law in a life-threatening situation, often at first contact and in a crisis. Or a very depressed and seriously dehydrated patient refusing all fluids could justifiably be given intravenous diazepam or even electroconvulsive therapy (ECT) forthwith to get drinking started again. Where a patient is already detained, section 62 of the MHA allows ECT to be given without MHAC prior approval in an emergency, for instance where the risk of suicide is very high. In practice, this usually means the first ECT only is given as, by the second, a

SOAD consultant will have assessed the patient. The keeping of full written records of what is being done at all times is an important additional safeguard. The patient's relatives should also be kept fully informed; it is hoped they will concur in the treatment, but their approval is not needed, and they cannot bar it.

The treatments controlled by the MHA and discussed here are ECT, psychotropic drugs, and the surgical implantation of sex hormones to reduce male sex drive. Leucotomy, a purely surgical procedure, is also controlled but is outside the scope of this book.

Electroconvulsive therapy

It is the responsibility of the doctor (not a nurse) to explain to the patient and relative why the treatment is necessary, how it is given, and the effects expected. This should be done in all cases, even where there is doubt whether the patient can understand, or is refusing. The doctor signs a form to say he has explained, and the patient signs, or refuses to, in which case this is noted. A record should also be made about the assessment of the patient's competence. When a detained patient gives consent, a special form is signed by the consultant stating the patient is in a fit state to make a decision and has agreed.

If the patient consents, it permits a course of treatments. Fresh consent will be needed for any further series and particularly if treatment is to be resumed after a gap of at least 21 days. The patient may at any time withdraw consent, and treatment then stops.

If the patient is uncertain about consenting, respect this uncertainty and leave the matter a while. Try again later: when they see they are not to be forced, and appreciate that ECT may be a rapid road to recovery and to leaving hospital, they may agree.

If the patient is incompetent to consent, or refuses to agree, and ECT is clearly needed, he/she must be detained if not already so and approval for ECT sought from the

SOAD consultant (section 53(3)(b)). The patient is required to be on a section 3 of the MHA as this clearly covers treatment but, as noted above, once the patient is well it can be cancelled. The case should also be discussed with the ECT team (anaesthetist and nurses) so that they know how important the treatment is, and how far to go with a seemingly unwilling patient.

Most patients will go along with treatment once all the paperwork has been done. It is a mistake to fight in the ECT room with a patient still determined to refuse. This should not arise if matters have been explained in a friendly way all along, particularly if a known nurse or doctor accompanies the patient to the ECT room and can talk with them encouragingly. Occasionally sedation before treatment (e.g. diazepam 2 mg orally) may be helpful, although benzodiazepines (including hypnotics) are best avoided since they shorten seizure time.

More detailed and useful information is contained in the report by the ECT Subcommittee of the Research Committee, Royal College of Psychiatrists (1989).

Drugs

Drugs may be given without the patient's consent if the patient is detained. After three months' treatment under section 3 of the MHA the responsible medical officer must sign a certificate that the patient understands the nature, purpose and effects of the drug and agrees to continue. Otherwise a second opinion must be obtained from a SOAD consultant (sections 58(1)(b) and (3)(b)). Long-stay in-patients may agree to treatment without understanding, so it is wise to have a documented second opinion, as above, if there is the slightest doubt.

Surgical implantation of hormones (but not of drugs) to reduce sex drive requires for all patients, whether detained or not, the patient's agreement; a doctor and two non-medical persons, all members of the MHAC, must certify that the patient understands and agrees to the treatment, and the doctor certifies that it should be given (section 57).

Out-patients

Patients on section 3 or 37 may be placed on trial leave (section 17) for a period usually of one to three months, with the taking of medication as part of the auditions of leave. This can only be continued until the Treatment Order expires.

Informal patients discharged on successful treatment with psychotropic drugs, including depot injections, may continue willingly with them thereafter if only because of a good relationship with the staff and/or as part of some continuing programme of social treatment. A few do not, however, and they may relapse and have to be readmitted. It is illegal to try to prevent relapse using drugs with a non-consenting informal patient. They can have no further treatment against their wishes unless their condition warrants a section of the MHA (usually section 3) and they are readmitted. Grounds for recommending this, besides the features of mental illness, include preventing further serious deterioration in the patient's health as well as dangerousness. A Guardianship Order (sections 7 and 8) can require a patient to attend for treatment but does not authorise any treatment, including drugs, against the patient's wishes. A Probation Order with a condition of treatment imposed by a court similarly does not compel the acceptance of medication.

Likewise, the Supervision and Treatment Orders introduced by the Criminal Procedures (Insanity and Unfitness to Plead) Act 1991, which provides more flexible disposal by courts of offenders found unfit to plead or not guilty by reason of insanity, are based on agreed treatment and supportive programmes on a voluntary basis. Thus, if the client refuses medication at a later date, it cannot be imposed.

Restriction Orders (section 37/41 of MHA) imposed by the courts when patients, if untreated, are considered a likely serious danger to the public, allow for longer-term treatment when they are 'on leave' in the community. If the patient no longer complies with medication, the Home

Office (which controls the patient's whereabouts) usually orders his/her return to hospital. When restricted patients are given a conditional discharge from their section by a Mental Health Tribunal, it is now usual to incorporate a 'long-term' plan of management, supervision and, where appropriate, long-term medication as part of the process.

Consent to physical examination and treatment by the mentally disordered is not covered by the MHA, whether patients are detained or informal. MHA sections apply to treatment for mental disorder only. But such patients, who may be unwilling or incapable of agreeing to necessary physical procedures, have a common law right to be treated appropriately. The medical and surgical treatment must be 'in the best interests of the patient' and, by implication, to preserve life, health and well-being. Full consultation (with relatives, the multidisciplinary team, specialists) is required and most hospitals now have clear guidelines with proper documentation to record that the necessary steps have been followed.

The procedures outlined above apply to England and Wales. Very similar practices are followed in the rest of the UK.

Reference

ECT Subcommittee of the Research Committee (1989) *The Practical Administration of Electroconvulsive Therapy*. London: Gaskell.

Appendix 2. Electroconvulsive treatment and abreaction

A series of induced epileptic fits, spaced out at two- or three-day intervals, is an effective treatment for serious depressive illness. Given more frequently, electroconvulsive therapy (ECT) suppresses mania, and one or two fits are enough to abolish catatonic stupor. It may be uniquely effective in puerperal psychosis. Combined with a phenothiazine it can be more effective in schizophrenia in the short-term than phenothiazine by itself (see p. 104). Why fits are therapeutic is unknown. It is simply an observed fact of human biology; but fits induce neuroendocine release and changes in the sensitivity of transmitter receptors in animals.

It is the fit and not the electricity of ECT which is the primary agent, because fits from an intravenous drug like 'Metrazol' or an inhaled vapour – hexafluorodiethyl ether or 'Indoklon' – are also therapeutic. Stimulation of a fit by brief pulses of current to the head is least unpleasant to the patient and most easily controlled. But there is evidence that the size and character of the pulse (of electricity) may matter too, whereas the duration of fit probably does not. Cognitive effects after ECT are related to the amount of electricity administered. The tonic and clonic muscle contractions of a convulsion are unnecessary (and if violent may result in fractures) so they are suppressed by giving a small dose of a muscle relaxant or paralyser acting at the motor end-plates. Commonly succinyl choline is used; it is normally quickly destroyed by a pseudocholine-esterase in the blood, so its action is brief. It is usually given under cover of anaesthesia with a short-acting intravenous barbiturate (methohexitone 0.75 mg/kg).

For therapeutic effect the fit must be bilateral and major in type, but what matters is the epileptic disturbance in the brain. Twitching of both thumbs and both big toes is simply an indicator to the operator that a major fit is occurring.

A useful technique (Hamilton Cuff technique) is to apply a sphygmomanometer cuff to one arm (the same side if using the unilateral electrodes) and block arterial blood flow (above systolic blood pressure). This is done before giving the intravenous drugs in the other arm, so that muscles distal to the cuff cannot receive relaxant. They can thus contract rhythmically when the epileptic discharge begins, even though the fit would be otherwise invisible because of the complete paralysis of the rest of the body muscles produced by the relaxant.

The treatment is physically safe, can be given to the very old, the frail, the pregnant, those with hypertension, cardiac arrhythmia, cardiac failure, Parkinson's disease, previous stroke or myocardial infarction (the last two 12 weeks or more after the attack). Since ECT with relaxant still produces brief marked rises in blood pressure, patients with aneurysms, recent cerebral haemorrhage or raised intracranial pressure should be regarded with very great caution, and avoided if possible.

The patient should be assessed the day after each treatment. In depressive illness there may be no change until after the first two or three treatments, when some improvement suddenly appears, and six or eight in all may be enough. Never give fixed courses. It is usual to give two more treatments when the patient is much improved. Patients differ. The elderly and brain-damaged are more likely to suffer memory disturbance. Too much ECT may result in hypomania, an acute brain syndrome, or restless anxiety. Fortunately these usually clear in 7–10 days and without additional medication. In schizophrenia a longer series of treatments, perhaps up to 12, may sometimes be needed.

Procedure

Explain the treatment to patient and relative, and get the necessary forms signed as evidence of consent. (See Appendix 1 – Consent to treatment.)

Discuss with the ECT team beforehand if there are any problems about consent and with the anaesthetist about any medical condition of the patient and about drugs already being taken (especially MAOIs which affect resuscitative measures). Benzodiazepines should be avoided as far as possible as they raise the seizure threshold.

Check the patient's dental state. False teeth should be removed before treatment, but decayed teeth may break in a fit and a piece be inhaled, so dental care beforehand may be indicated.

As before any general anaesthetic, the patient fasts overnight, but may have a cup of tea three hours beforehand. Diabetics require special arrangements: they will continue with regular insulin and glucose and have their ECT at a conveniently-timed appointment.

The hair must be free from grease and lacquer and the skin clean, to make good electrical contact with the electrodes. All metal objects (hair slide, glasses) must be removed to avoid short-circuits.

If the patient has a cold or respiratory infection on treatment morning, treatment must be postponed for another day. A nervous or doubtful patient may be encouraged by the presence and supportive conversation of a nurse or doctor he/she knows.

The treatment is given to each patient, singly, in a separate room with the door closed. The sight or the sound of a person receiving ECT and the comments of the ECT team can alarm those waiting. Separate waiting, treatment and recovery rooms are recommended.

Before the patient comes into the treatment room, make yourself familiar with the ECT machine and its calibration. Examine the patient's ECT form, which ought to show information relevant to giving anaesthetic and ECT, in particular drug treatment and medical conditions.

The notes of previous ECT will show:

(a)   the doses of muscle relaxant and anaesthetic previously used and whether effective

(b)   the setting on the ECT machine which gave a fit

(c)   the non-dominant side if the patient is to have unilateral ECT

(d)   problems such as difficulty in finding a vein, failure to get a fit, or prolonged apnoea.

Fresh entries are made after each treatment.

The patient receives, from the anaesthetist, the anaesthetic and relaxant and, when unconscious, a few squeezes of oxygen from the re-breathing bag. A gag is then placed between the teeth to protect the tongue. The relaxant causes muscles to fasciculate. Wait a few moments for this to die away.

The electrodes are then applied to the head, either one on each side (bilateral) or both on the same side (unilateral), the non-dominant side of the cerebrum (see Fig. 9). The

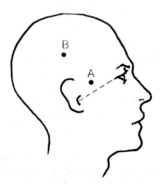

Fig. 9   Unilateral ECT: electrodes are placed (A) 4 cm above midpoint between earhole and angle of eye; and (B) 6 cm from A, above ear

first is technically a little easier and slightly more effective, the second has the advantage of quicker recovery after the fit and far less risk of memory disturbance. But which is the non-dominant side? In right-handed people, and in two-thirds of left-handed or ambidextrous people, it is the right side of the head; in the rest it is the left side. Asking about or testing for hand, foot and eye preference usually shows dominance. Otherwise, give the first unilateral treatment to the left side and the second to the right side, and compare the after-effects; continue treatments on the side causing less memory disturbance.

The electrodes must be well moistened to conduct evenly, otherwise the current may not pass or may cause a skin burn. On the other hand, if they are very wet, fluid will run on the skin and may allow a short circuit. Press them firmly into the cleansed skin with a slight twist and hold them there until the fit is over. Recent work indicates that electrodes applied bifrontally, that is 5 cm above the external angle of orbit on each side, produces fits more effectively than when applied unilaterally, but with a similar lack of memory disturbance.

Press the ECT button. The immediate tonic muscular contraction is a direct response to the current and not a fit. But after about 10 seconds, or longer, a rhythmic jerking begins in the eyelids, thumbs and toes. It dies away after about 40 seconds and the patient lies relaxed and apnoeic. Movement must be bilaterally symmetrical, even with unilateral stimulation, to be a sign of an effective fit. The recommended duration of fits is 20–50 seconds.

Although there is no clear relationship between duration of seizure and effectiveness of treatment, fits longer than one minute are associated with more confusion and memory loss.

If no fit has occurred, repeat the stimulation once at a much higher electrical setting. Induced hyperventilation by the anaesthetist can help to lower the seizure threshold. If this fails, postpone a fresh try to another day. Each electric shock adds to the side-effects.

Thresholds for fits vary. The threshold is raised by drugs with anticonvulsant properties, such as benzodiazepines, the anaesthetic agent propofol, or high doses of methohexitone (more than 1.5 mg/kg). Dry electrodes, dirty skin, and oily hair can insulate from the electric shock and cause fit failure with an apparently satisfactory setting.

When the fit is over, oxygen is given after inserting an airway. Shortly afterwards the patient begins to breathe. After the resumption of spontaneous breathing the patient is turned on one side and transferred to a recovery room for post-anaesthetic care. A nurse must be present until consciousness returns and post-fit confusion settled enough for the patient to be safe alone.

Recovery of spontaneous breathing is sometimes delayed. Artificial respiration will then have to be continued. Delayed recovery beyond 30 minutes is an anaesthetic emergency requiring intubation and transfer to intensive care. Delay can result from too much muscle-relaxant, rarely because of pseudo-cholinesterase deficiency, an autosomal recessive condition. Recovery to consciousness takes a few minutes, the time depending on the anaesthetic drug and its dose, other sedative drugs, age and state of health.

Brief confusion, restlessness, headache and nausea are common following ECT. A cup of tea, a lie-down and an aspirin may help these after-effects disappear. Assessment for therapeutic benefit should be made the next day, after each treatment. Amnesia for events immediately before ECT (anterograde) and patchy losses of memory after ECT (retrograde amnesia), most often for less important matters, is common. Memory difficulties usually subside in two or three weeks but may persist for longer. Depressive illness does itself appear to be associated with memory impairment and distinguishing between this and an ECT effect may be impossible.

ECT is a medical treatment given for serious mental illness. Ultimately the psychiatrist must balance the need for ECT against the risks of giving ECT and then decide in consultation with the anaesthetist whether to give it and under what circumstances.

Abreaction

A dose of anaesthetic insufficient to anaesthetise produces a state of altered consciousness, calm, relaxed, dreamy, inattentive to surroundings, and more suggestible. This state induces freer, less guarded speech and can be used as a diagnostic aid for mute states or as an adjunct to psychotherapy. The tecnhique has been called 'interview with sedation', or 'abreaction' when accompanied by the display of strong emotion.

Mute states not due to neurological or medical causes are usually hysterical fugues or psychoses. An interview with sedation may enable the diagnosis, the forgotten identity being recalled or abnormal psychotic experiences and thinking being revealed.

The discovery of delusions, abnormal thinking, or abnormal experiences thus allows appropriate treatment for a depressive illness or schizophrenia.

In fugue states the recollection of identity may be accompanied by remembrance of unpleasant events preceding the memory loss, with emotional display and subsequent improvement. Persons of previously good personality whose symptoms began following a distressing event – post-traumatic disorder for example – may re-experience the event. Emotions, allowed open expression and re-enactment, may lose their force, and clinical improvement may result.

A barbiturate or benzodiazepine by intravenous injection are the safest and easiest drugs to use. Sodium amytal (250 mg in 5 ml or 500 mg in 10 ml) is usually enough. The injection is commenced intravenously at the rate of 1 ml per minute while talking to the patient and noting respiration. Other drugs are 2.5% solution of sodium thiopentone, starting with 3 ml intravenously and then at the rate of 1 ml per minute up to 15 ml, or diazepam 10–20 mg intravenously over several minutes, although this tends to be less effective. It is best to have two doctors present, and an Ambu bag and oropharyngeal airway available, although these should not be required.

Talking may begin with suggestions of comfort and relaxation and asking about the effects of the injection; a heavy sigh is often the sign of the drug acting. Then proceed to ask about neutral matters of personal history before moving on to incidents or topics of emotional concern. Do not give more drug than necessary to reach the relaxed state or the patient may go into a long sleep and forget. If important memories are recalled, keep the patient talking until the drug effect wears off, so that the recollection is maintained in full consciousness.

After recovery from the drug, discussion of the material uncovered helps to re-establish and re-integrate the forgotten material.

Appendix 3. People who take overdoses

Self-poisoning, admitted or discovered, raises the questions of future suicide (to be prevented), or life stresses (to be alleviated) and of mental illness (to be treated). All people who take overdoses require assessment from these three points of view. Resuscitation and treatment of toxicity is a medical matter, perhaps in an accident or emergency centre or a medical ward, and comes first. Psychiatric assessment should begin there as early as possible. Bear in mind the following and cover all points.

(a) Some patients claim the overdose was an accident, or taken only to get some sleep and without lethal intent. It is dangerous to accept this at face value: they should be assessed like all other overdoses.

(b) Unless the patient works with drugs, he/she is likely to have some mistaken ideas of what is dangerous and the actual dose of drug is an unreliable guide to assess the degree of suicidal intent. Someone who takes only very few tablets may firmly intend death. Additionally, mental illness causes indecision with sudden reversals of action and resulting in incomplete dosing. All who have taken anything should be assessed.

(c) Overdosers all have a set of individual problems but it is useful to classify them into groups which provide guidelines as to further management:

(i)   Those who have a significant mental illness with either persistent or recurrent ideas of death-intent but who fail through accident, insufficient knowledge or indecision. If the illness is untreated, they are likely to try again.

(ii)   A few who use suicidal threats and acts to gain enjoyable dramatic attention or to manipulate relatives, doctors and others.

(iii)   Some who attempt suicide as a result of social pressures such as difficulties in relationships, business failure and financial ruin, marital breakup with custody battles and money problems.

(iv)   Those who were not thinking positively of death but trying to escape from some seemingly hopeless situation, to let fate decide the future or to test the attitudes of others.

(d) Group (i) carry a high risk of suicide, sooner or later, and should have psychiatric care, probably as in-patients. Compulsory admission under a section of the Mental Health Act (MHA) should be considered if the patient is unwilling to cooperate. Group (ii) pose a special problem in that, strictly, they are not mentally ill but tend to repeat the pattern while the response is gratifying, a dangerous practice which could be lethal. Group (iii) is particularly difficult as, if there are no signs of mental illness, help can only be offered on a voluntary basis and the very real problems that lead to overdose may persist.

(e) The initial assessment is to decide the presence of significant mental illness, usually a depressive one, but schizophrenics, too, plan to kill themselves when overwhelmed by distressing symptoms or an alien world. Thus, the mental state is explored gauging the severity of morbidness, fears and preoccupations. Biological changes of insomnia, weight loss, lack of energy and concentration help to indicate the severity and persistence of the illness. Personality is very relevant in all overdoses – whether impulsive or a planner, a loner or gregarious, intelligent or not, rigid or open to suggestion. Always check for excessive alcohol intake, a potent factor in overdosage and suicide. Thus a systematic medical and psychiatric history and mental state is needed along with details of the attempt.

(f) Information, whether the patient is accessible or not, should also be obtained from a relative or friend, not only for general history but to explore sensitive areas such as alcohol intake or drug abuse. Ask, too, in detail about the overdose, for example how secret was it, how impulsive or planned? Had the patient's behaviour changed in the previous day or so? Are social/interpersonal stresses as severe as the patient perceives them?

(g) The environmental and emotional stresses the patient has recently experienced are especially relevant to group (c)(iii). While the clinician may readily sympathise with, for example, a disastrous marriage or catastrophic loss of job, it may lead to an underestimate of suicidal risk. 'Understanding' the basis for the patient's act can lead to empathy but confuses the issue of risk. What matters is the patient's vulnerability as at present shown by current symptoms and recent behaviour and the immediate need to prevent further self-damage. General pointers to high risk such as previous serious attempts, being male, intractable physical illness, living alone, loss of partner, unemployment and old age should be given due weight. Drug and alcohol abuse are particularly relevant.

(h) A small diagnostic problem arises with patients who have for long been chronic surgery attenders, with insomnia of some degree, anxiety, psychosomatic symptoms or hypochondriacal complaints. A more serious acute depression may have quietly emerged, but may not be recognised except by inquiring for new symptoms, including those of a biological nature. If not, the wrong assumpton of a continued mild neuroticism will be made. Everlasting complainers unable to accept help but continuing to complain may turn to suicide when they see everyone is exhausted and no longer tolerant of them.

(i) Having judged any further suicidal risk and relevance of mental illness and social factors, the clinician needs to decide on a plan of help. Always be ready to consult with senior or other colleagues, if uncertain what to do. The clearly mentally ill who remain at risk usually need hospital psychiatric treatment, possibly under compulsion using a section of the MHA. But more often treatment continues at home and then a reliable network of carers and appropriate drug treatment needs to be set up and monitored. For those not mentally ill and with seemingly hopeless personal problems, the task is more difficult. Usually, use of the MHA is inappropriate and the psychiatrist will need all his therapeutic skill to persuade the patient to accept help from professionals and other carers. Establishing a thin line of confidence between the patient and therapist may just turn a black situation into something lighter. It requires commitment and continuity, with a realistic appraisal of difficulties and possible solutions. Social work may alter some of the stresses, supportive psychotherapy increase toleration and, in the longer term, cognitive and interpersonal therapy alter perception and increase confidence. The overdose, itself, may produce changes, a signal to relatives and friends to rally round.

(j) For those who are discharged home and remain at risk, the further care plan should be recorded in the notes. Identify who is the key professional worker to provide further contact and continuity, for example community nurse or therapist, hospital doctor, general practitioner, or social worker. Clear communications with and between them and the patient's family is essential.

(k) Assessment of overdosers can be haphazard in general hospitals, perhaps not done at all, or done by junior staff without psychiatric experience. One consultant psychiatrist should be responsible for setting up a service to provide systematic assessment of suicide in accident and emergency or medical wards. Assessment can be by nurses, social workers or junior doctors provided the consultant ensures they receive essential training. Weekly reviews with a senior doctor are good practice. Regular refresher sessions are required and systematic data collection helps maintain standards. This also provides a basis for clinical audit along with reviews of any later successful suicides.

Appendix 4. Other sources of information

More detailed and invaluable up-to-date information on the clinical use and cost of drugs is contained in the *British National Formulary* (BNF), published by the British Medical Association and the Royal Pharmaceutical Society of Great Britain twice a year, and issued regularly to medical practitioners. It also provides the telephone numbers of drug information services and for the emergency treatment of poisoning. There is general guidance on prescribing and more specific details for prescribing controlled drugs. Regulations are altered from time-to-time and it is important to check the up-to-date rules by referring to the most recent BNF. The BNF is also a valuable source on possible drug interaction.

The *Monthly Index of Medical Specialities* (MIMS), published by Haymarket Publishing Ltd, London, also gives lists of drugs and their costs but with limited information on clinical use.

The *Data Sheet Compendium* of the Association of the British Pharmaceutical Industry (ABPI) contains detailed information for doctors from the manufacturers about individual drugs. It is revised annually.

Further reading

AYD, F. J. & BLACKWELL, B. (1984) *Discoveries in Biological Psychiatry.* New York: Ayd Medical Community.

DAVIES, D. M. (ed.) (1991) *Textbook of Adverse Drug Reactions* (4th edn). Oxford: Oxford University Press.

DUKES, M. N. G. (ed.) (1988) *Meyler's Side Effects of Drugs* (11th edn). Amsterdam: Elsevier.

GILMAN, A. G., *et al* (1985) *The Pharmacological Basis of Therapeutics* (7th edn). New York: Macmillan.

MELTZER, H. Y. (ed.) (1987) *Psychopharmacology: A Third Generation of Progress.* New York: Raven Press.

Index 1. Names of drugs
Compiled by Linda English

The proprietary or trade names are given in italics; the page numbers for the main entries are shown in bold type.

Index 2. Symptoms and usages

Compiled by Linda English

The page numbers for the main entries are shown in bold type.